# Concise Anatomy
# for Anaesthesia

# Concise Anatomy
# for Anaesthesia

**Andreas G Erdmann**

Fellow in Pain Management
London
Specialist Registrar in Anaesthesia
East Anglian Deanery

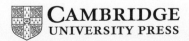

CAMBRIDGE
UNIVERSITY PRESS

CAMBRIDGE UNIVERSITY PRESS
Cambridge, New York, Melbourne, Madrid, Cape Town, Singapore, São Paulo

Cambridge University Press
The Edinburgh Building, Cambridge CB2 8RU, UK

Published in the United States of America by Cambridge University Press, New York

www.cambridge.org
Information on this title: www.cambridge.org/9780521869096

First published 2002
Reprinted by Cambridge University Press 2006
Reprinted 2007

Printed in the United Kingdom at the University Press, Cambridge

ISBN 978-0-521-86909-6 hardback

# Contents

# Foreword

When I first started my anaesthesia job, it did not take me long to realise that I was going to have to relearn a lot of anatomy that had been implanted in my short-term memory during the second MB. I was, incorrectly, under the impression that anatomy was the sole preserve of the surgeon.

From the moment that a career in anaesthesia is started, anatomy plays a part. Dr Andreas Erdmann decided to write this book following his experiences during the final FRCA examination. The idea is a simple one, combining simple line diagrams and succinct text to cover all of the areas of anatomy essential to modern anaesthetic practice. It will be invaluable as a revision text for the FRCA, but will also help anaesthetists to retain anatomy knowledge throughout their careers. It will be useful for consultants teaching trainees and also for other theatre personnel to understand the procedures carried out by anaesthetists.

I am sure that generations of anaesthetists will be grateful to Dr Erdmann for providing such a simple and comprehensive review of an essential subject.

Richard Griffiths MD FRCA
*Peterborough, June 2001*

# Preface

The origin of this concise book of anatomy results from many comments from FRCA examination candidates. Anatomy has always played an important role in the examination syllabus, as well as being of great practical importance in the everyday practice of anaesthesia. It is also a subject that appears to demand a disproportionately large amount of time during examination preparation. However, neglect of the anatomical subject-matter is perilous and leads to the loss of valuable 'easy' marks.

The idea behind this book is to present a concise and easily digestible outline of anatomy that has been extensively based on the current FRCA examination syllabus. I have attempted to present the core anatomical knowledge required for the Primary and Final FRCA examinations in a simple and straightforward manner. There are numerous diagrams to illustrate the subject matter, as well as additional space for the addition of personal notes. It is, however, impossible within the constraints of this book to provide in-depth detail and this should be obtained by reference to some of the larger textbooks. Sample questions are included at the end of each section, and include questions similar to those asked in previous examinations.

It is hoped that this book may also be of help to those teaching anatomy to FRCA candidates, as well as to all practising anaesthetists wishing to 'brush up' on some forgotten anatomical detail. Nurses, operating theatre practitioners and other healthcare professionals will also find this book of use when gaining a practical understanding of applied anatomy.

Finally, all errors and omissions are my responsibility, and any comments and advice for improvement will be gratefully accepted.

Andreas Erdmann
*June 2001*

# Respiratory
# System

# I   The mouth

## DESCRIPTION

The mouth extends from the lips (anterior) to the isthmus of the fauces (posterior). There are two sections:

> Vestibule – slit-like cavity between the cheeks/lips and gingivae/teeth
> Oral cavity – from the teeth to the oropharyngeal isthmus

## RELATIONS

Roof – hard and soft palate
Floor – tongue and reflection of the gum mucous membrane
Posterior – isthmus separates the oral cavity from the oropharynx

## POINTS OF INTEREST

- Papilla – a papilla for the opening of the parotid duct is present on the cheek opposite the upper second molar tooth
- Midline frenulum – under the tongue, has two papillae for the submandibular duct openings and the sublingual fold (of mucous membrane) for numerous tiny sublingual duct openings
- Isthmus – contains three structures: the palatoglossal folds (anterior), the palatine tonsils (middle) and the palatopharyngeal folds (posterior). It is bounded by the soft palate above
- Hard palate – created by the maxilla (palatine process) anteriorly and palatine bone posteriorly
- Soft palate – a suspended 'curtain' from the hard palate with a midline uvula; a fibrous palatine aponeurosis forms the skeleton of the soft palate

## VASCULAR SUPPLY

1. Vestibule – facial artery (via superior and inferior labial branches)
2. Teeth – maxillary artery (via superior and inferior alveolar branches)
3. Tongue – lingual artery (venous via lingual vein into internal jugular)
4. Palate – mixed supply from facial, maxillary and ascending pharyngeal arteries

## NERVE SUPPLY

- Vestibule:
  - Sensory from the branches of the trigeminal nerve (V2 and V3)
  - Motor from the facial nerve (VII)
- Tongue:
  - Taste – anterior two-thirds via the facial nerve (VII via chorda tympani), posterior one-third via the glossopharyngeal nerve (IX)
  - Motor from the hypoglossal nerve (XII)
- Palate:
  - Sensory and motor from the trigeminal nerve (V2)
  - Taste from the facial nerve

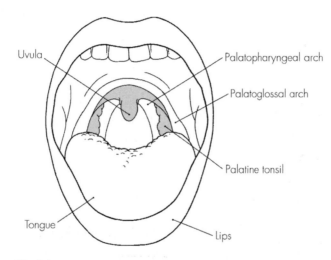

Uvula

Palatopharyngeal arch

Palatoglossal arch

Palatine tonsil

Tongue

Lips

**Fig 1.1**
The mouth

# 2 The nose

## DESCRIPTION

A pyramidal structure of bone, cartilage and the nasal cavities. A midline nasal septum divides the nasal cavity into two separate areas, which open anteriorly via the nares and posteriorly via the choanae.

## RELATIONS

Roof – arch-like, nasal cartilages and nasal bones anteriorly, cribriform plate (of ethmoid) in the middle, and sphenoid and clivus (occipital) bones posteriorly

Floor – horizontal plate of the palatine bone, palatine process of the maxilla

Medial wall – nasal septum (cartilage and ethmoid/vomer)

Lateral wall – bony framework (ethmoid/maxilla/palatine bone) and bony conchae (superior, middle and inferior)

## POINTS OF INTEREST

- Sinuses – drain into the nose interior via numerous openings. Above the superior concha lies the spheno-ethmoidal recess, which drains the sphenoidal sinus. Below the superior concha lies the superior meatus, draining the posterior ethmoidal air cells. Respectively below each concha lie the middle meatus (draining ethmoidal, maxillary and frontal sinuses) and the inferior meatus, which drains the nasolacrimal duct and tears from the eye
- Nose – lined by mucoperiosteum (highly vascular)

## VASCULAR SUPPLY

1. Ophthalmic (anterior and posterior ethmoidal branches) and maxillary (sphenopalatine branch) arteries
2. Venous drainage via the facial vein to the internal jugular vein

## NERVE SUPPLY

- Olfactory nerve (I) to the olfactory zone
- Trigeminal nerve (V1 and V2), with multiple sensory branches to the entire nose

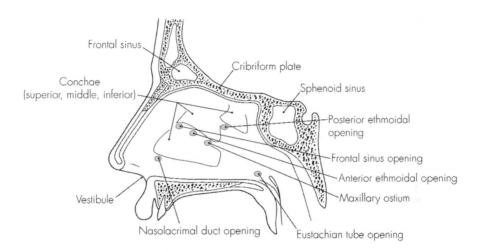

**Fig 2.1**
The nose

# 3   The pharynx

## DESCRIPTION

A midline muscular tube that provides a common pathway for the ingestion of food and for respiration. It arises from the base of skull and ends at C6. It is divided into three sections: naso-, oro- and laryngopharynx. The wall has four layers: mucosa, submucosa (tough fascia), muscular and loose connective tissue.

## RELATIONS

Anterior – nose and mouth

Posterior – retropharyngeal space, prevertebral fascia and upper six cervical vertebrae

Superior – sphenoid (body) and occipital (basilar region) bones

Inferior – becomes continuous with the oesophagus

## POINTS OF INTEREST

- Two groups of muscles:
  - Constrictors – three paired muscles: inferior, middle and superior constrictors
  - Elevators – stylopharyngeus, salpingopharyngeus and palatopharyngeus
- Swallowing:
  - Phase 1 – food bolus is pushed towards the oropharynx by the tongue
  - Phase 2 – respiration is halted, the oropharynx and nasopharynx close, the larynx is elevated, constricted and pushed forward, and the bolus passes over (protective) the epiglottis into the pharynx. Constrictor muscles ensure the consecutive propulsion into the oesophagus
  - Phase 3 – once it is in the oesophagus, peristaltic waves ensure the progression of the bolus to the stomach

## VASCULAR SUPPLY

1. Arterial – ascending pharyngeal, facial, maxillary, lingual (to epiglottis) and both thyroid arteries
2. Venous – via the pharyngeal plexus to the internal jugular vein

## NERVE SUPPLY

- From pharyngeal plexus:
  - Sensory – pharyngeal branches of glossopharyngeal (IX) and vagus (X) nerves
  - Motor – vagus via the pharyngeal plexus (except stylopharyngeus – IX)

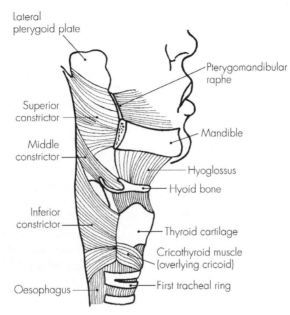

Lateral
pterygoid plate

Pterygomandibular
raphe

Superior
constrictor

Mandible

Middle
constrictor

Hyoglossus

Hyoid bone

Inferior
constrictor

Thyroid cartilage

Cricothyroid muscle
(overlying cricoid)

Oesophagus

First tracheal ring

**Fig 3.1**
The pharynx

# 4    The larynx

## DESCRIPTION

The larynx forms a functional protective sphincter of the respiratory tract as well as containing the vocal apparatus. It consists of a complex arrangement of muscles, cartilage, membranes and ligaments. It extends from C3 to C6 in the midline (adult).

## RELATIONS

Anterior – superficial structure, is covered by the fascia (deep and superficial), platysma and skin
Posterior – pharynx, prevertebral muscles and cervical vertebrae
Superior – pharynx
Inferior – becomes continuous with the trachea

## STRUCTURE

1.  Hyoid bone (at C3) – not strictly part of the larynx but firmly attached above it
2.  Cartilages (nine) – three unpaired and six paired:
    *   Epiglottis (elastic) – 'leaf'-shaped; the lower, narrower end is attached to the thyroid cartilage by the thyro-epiglottic ligament, and the upper broader end is free to project superiorly
    *   Thyroid cartilage (hyaline) – like a 'shield'. It is the largest of the laryngeal cartilages and a midline structure. Upper (at C4) and lower (at C5) borders carry cornua (horns) posteriorly – inferior

cornu also has a facet for articulation with the cricoid cartilage
*   Cricoid cartilage (hyaline) – 'signet ring'-shaped and situated at the C6 level. It articulates on its lateral border with the thyroid cornua, and on its upper border with the arytenoid cartilages (paired)
*   Arytenoid cartilages (paired) – pyramidal in shape, each with a lateral muscular process (for insertion of both crico-arytenoid muscles) and an anterior vocal process (being the posterior attachment of the vocal ligament)
*   Corniculate cartilages (paired) and cuneiform cartilages (paired) – these provide attachments for some intrinsic laryngeal muscles and are both found within the aryepiglottic folds (the fibro-elastic membrane between the epiglottis and arytenoids – lower border of which is free and forms the vestibular ligament or false cord)

3.  Ligaments – four extrinsic and minor intrinsic (small synovial capsules):
    *   Thyrohyoid membrane – between the upper border of the thyroid and the hyoid bone. Strengthened anteriorly and laterally
    *   Hyo-epiglottic ligament – connects the hyoid bone to the lower part of the epiglottis
    *   Cricothyroid ligament – between the thyroid above and the cricoid below, the preferred site for cricothyrotomy

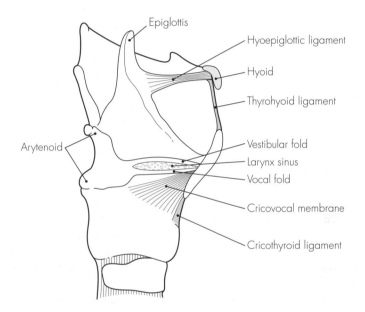

Epiglottis

Hyoepiglottic ligament

Hyoid

Thyrohyoid ligament

Vestibular fold

Larynx sinus

Vocal fold

Cricovocal membrane

Cricothyroid ligament

Arytenoid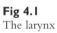

**Fig 4.1**
The larynx

- Cricotracheal ligament – connects the cricoid to the first ring of the trachea
4. Muscles – three extrinsic (connect larynx to its neighbours) and six intrinsic:
   - Extrinsic:
     - Sternothyroid – depresses the larynx, connects the posterior manubrium sterni to the lateral thyroid lamina
     - Thyrohyoid – elevates the larynx, connects the lateral thyroid lamina to the inferior greater horn of the hyoid bone
     - Inferior constrictor – constricts the pharynx, origins from the thyroid lamina, the tendinous arch over the cricothyroid and the side of the pharynx
   - Intrinsic:
     - Posterior crico-arytenoid – opens the glottis by the abducting cords
     - Lateral crico-arytenoid – closes the glottis by the adducting cords
     - Interarytenoid (unpaired) – closes the glottis (especially posteriorly) by connecting the arytenoids. Some fibres become the aryepiglottic muscle laterally, which constricts the laryngeal inlet somewhat
     - Thyro-arytenoid – relaxes the cords by shortening, thus pulling the arytenoids anteriorly
     - Vocalis – fine adjustment of vocal cord tension (fibres come from the thyro-arytenoid)
     - Cricothyroid – only true tensor and the only muscle that lies outside the cartilages. It works by tilting the cricoid and putting stretch on the vocal cords

## POINTS OF INTEREST

- Laryngeal nerve injuries:
  - External branch of the superior laryngeal nerve is in close association with the superior thyroid vessels and may be damaged during surgery. As the cricothyroid is the only muscle supplied, there is loss of cord tension and hoarseness following unilateral damage. This is frequently temporary as the opposite cricothyroid compensates
  - Recurrent laryngeal nerve is in close association with the inferior thyroid vessels and the lower lobe of thyroid, and may also be damaged during thyroidectomy. In addition, an enlarged thyroid gland, lymph nodes or cervical trauma may involve the recurrent laryngeal nerve. On the left side the thoracic course of the nerve puts it at risk from malignant lung, oesophageal or lymph node tumours, and even from aortic aneurysms or an enlarged right atrium. Such injury results in a paralysed (cadaveric) midline vocal cord position – and hoarseness if unilateral, which usually resolves following opposite cord over-activity. However, bilateral nerve injury results in total loss of vocal cord function and the resultant flap-like valve effect can result in severe stridor and dyspnoea
- Local anaesthesia of the airway is imperative for awake fibreoptic intubation. The simplest method is to use nebulised lignocaine to anaesthetise the whole airway, but this is probably the least effective method. Local anaesthetic may be applied to the nose, mouth and pharynx, and a spray-as-you-go

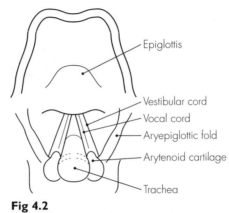

**Fig 4.2**
The larynx (view at laryngoscopy)

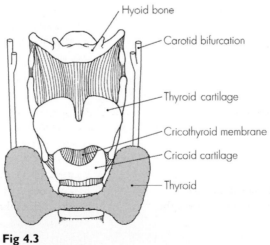

**Fig 4.3**
Laryngeal structures

technique is used (under direct vision) for the laryngeal structures. This can be supplemented by a cricothyroid membrane puncture with an intratracheal spray of local anaesthetic. Individual blockade of the external branch of the superior laryngeal nerve (at the greater horn of the hyoid) and of its internal branch (in the piriform fossa) has been arguably superseded by the prior methods

## VASCULAR SUPPLY

1. Arterial:
   - Superior laryngeal (from superior thyroid artery) – accompanies the internal branch of the superior laryngeal nerve
   - Inferior laryngeal (from inferior thyroid artery) – accompanies the recurrent laryngeal nerve
2. Venous – into the corresponding superior and inferior thyroid veins

## NERVE SUPPLY

- Branches of vagus (X) nerve:
  - Superior laryngeal nerve – passes deep to the internal and external carotid arteries and then divides into:
    External branch (small) – motor to cricothyroid
    Internal branch (larger) – sensory above the vocal cords and the inferior surface of the epiglottis (superior surface of the epiglottis is supplied by the glossopharyngeal nerve)
- Recurrent (inferior) laryngeal nerve – on the right side it leaves the vagus as it crosses the subclavian artery, loops under it and ascends in the tracheo-oesophageal groove. On the left side it leaves the vagus as it crosses the aortic arch, loops under it and ascends in the tracheo-oesophageal groove. It supplies:
  Motor to all intrinsic muscles of the larynx (except cricothyroid)
  Sensation below the vocal cords

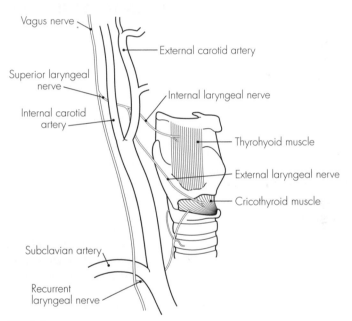

**Fig 4.4**
Nerve supply of the larynx

# 5    The trachea

## DESCRIPTION

It is a roughly midline structure that extends from C6 (at the lower edge of the cricoid cartilage) to the carinal bifurcation at T4. It is 15 cm long in the adult and has up to 20 C-shaped cartilages joined by fibro-elastic tissue that is deficient posteriorly. The trachealis muscle closes the posterior border.

## RELATIONS

In the neck:
   Anterior – skin, superficial and deep fascia, thyroid isthmus (over second to fourth rings), sternothyroid and sternohyoid muscles (lower neck) and the anterior jugular vein communications and thyroidea ima artery (also lower neck)
   Posterior – oesophagus and recurrent laryngeal nerves
   Laterally – lateral lobes of the thyroid and carotid sheath (with internal jugular vein, common carotid artery and vagus nerve)
In the thorax:
   Anterior (in caudad direction) – inferior thyroid veins, sternothyroid origins, thymus remnants, brachiocephalic artery, left common carotid artery and aortic arch. The pulmonary bifurcation lies behind the carina
   Posterior – oesophagus and left recurrent laryngeal nerve
   Laterally:
      • Right – pleura, azygos vein and right vagus nerve
      • Left – pleura, left common carotid, left subclavian artery, aortic arch and left vagus

## POINTS OF INTEREST

   • Tracheostomy:
      • Positioning – all important. With full extension of the head and neck it is achieved by using a sandbag under the patient's shoulders. Keeping strictly to the midline minimises the risk of major vessel damage. During formal tracheostomy the skin incision is deepened by blunt dissection, the thyroid isthmus is retracted or divided, and a window is opened in the trachea between the second and fourth rings. Higher placement may result in an increased incidence of tracheal stenosis. The largest tracheostomy tube for a comfortable fit is then inserted
      • Percutaneous techniques – require less dissection, but the same principle of keeping strictly to the midline also applies

## VASCULAR SUPPLY

1. Arterial – inferior thyroid arteries
2. Venous – inferior thyroid veins

## NERVE SUPPLY

   • Recurrent laryngeal branch of the vagus and sympathetic branches of the middle cervical ganglion

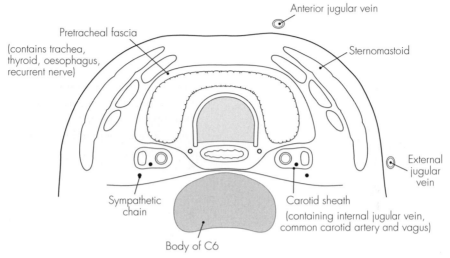

**Fig 5.1**
The trachea (cross-section)

Anterior jugular vein

Pretracheal fascia
(contains trachea,
thyroid, oesophagus,
recurrent nerve)

Sternomastoid

External
jugular
vein

Sympathetic
chain

Carotid sheath
(containing internal jugular vein,
common carotid artery and vagus)

Body of C6

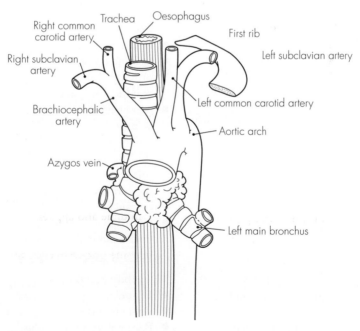

**Fig 5.2**
Relations of the trachea

Right common
carotid artery

Trachea   Oesophagus

First rib

Right subclavian
artery

Left subclavian artery

Brachiocephalic
artery

Left common carotid artery

Aortic arch

Azygos vein

Left main bronchus

# 6 The bronchi and bronchial tree

## DESCRIPTION

The trachea bifurcates at the T4 level into the right and left main bronchi. The last tracheal ring is wider and larger, and forms a ridge called the carina.

The right main bronchus is shorter, wider and more vertical than the left (25°). After 2.5 cm, it gives off the right upper bronchus. The left main bronchus is more angled (45°) and is 5 cm long.

## RELATIONS

Right main bronchus – passes under the azygos vein arch and lies above and then behind the right pulmonary artery

Left main bronchus – passes under the aortic arch, in front of the oesophagus, thoracic duct and descending aorta, and lies below and then behind the left pulmonary artery

## STRUCTURE

1. Right main bronchus terminates in three lobar bronchi – upper, middle and lower – that supply the respective lung lobes. Each lobar bronchus then terminates in segmental bronchi as follows:
   - Upper – apical, anterior and posterior
   - Middle – lateral and medial
   - Lower – superior, medial basal, anterior basal, lateral basal and posterior basal

2. Left main bronchus terminates in two lobar bronchi – upper and lower – also supplying the respective lung lobes. The corresponding segmental bronchi are:
   - Upper – apical, anterior, posterior, superior lingual and inferior lingual
   - Lower – superior, medial basal (small and variable), anterior basal, lateral basal and posterior basal

The layers of the bronchial wall are:
- Mucosa – with ciliated cells and goblet cells. In smaller bronchi, goblet cells become fewer. The alveoli are lined only with very thin epithelium
- Basement membrane
- Submucous layer – elastic fibres that provide elastic recoil to the air conduction system
- Muscular layer – unstriped and arranged to withstand pressures (geodesic framework). The relative thickness increases as bronchi get smaller – it acts as a sphincter beyond the terminal bronchioles (at the entrance to the alveolar ducts)
- Cartilage – rings are replaced by plates in the intrapulmonary bronchi and become progressively less complete

The subdivisions are:
- Bronchus
- Bronchiolus – cartilage disappears
- Respiratory bronchiolus
- Alveolar duct
- Alveolar sac
- Alveolus

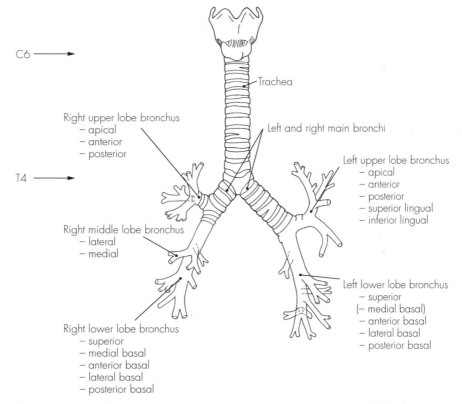

C6 ⟶

Trachea

Right upper lobe bronchus
  – apical
  – anterior
  – posterior

Left and right main bronchi

Left upper lobe bronchus
  – apical
  – anterior
  – posterior
  – superior lingual
  – inferior lingual

T4 ⟶

Right middle lobe bronchus
  – lateral
  – medial

Left lower lobe bronchus
  – superior
  (– medial basal)
  – anterior basal
  – lateral basal
  – posterior basal

Right lower lobe bronchus
  – superior
  – medial basal
  – anterior basal
  – lateral basal
  – posterior basal

**Fig 6.1**
The bronchial tree

# 7    The pleura and mediastinum

## DESCRIPTION

The lungs are enveloped in a twin-walled serous sac – two layers of the pleura – that meet at the hilum to form the pulmonary ligament. A potential space exists between the two pleural layers (visceral and parietal), which contains a thin film of serous fluid.

The mediastinum is the space between the two pleural sacs and is divided into four regions by the pericardium:

Superior (below thoracic inlet)
Middle (contains pericardial contents)
Anterior (behind sternum)
Posterior (above diaphragm)

## POINTS OF INTEREST

- Lines of pleural reflection (surface markings):
  - Apex – lies 4 cm above the clavicle
  - Behind the sternoclavicular joint
  - Behind the sternum at the second costochondral junction
  - On the left – lateral sternal edge at the fourth cartilage
  - On the right – down to the costoxiphoid angle
  - Eighth rib – mid-clavicular line
  - Tenth rib – mid-axillary line
  - Twelfth rib – posterior to the costovertebral angle

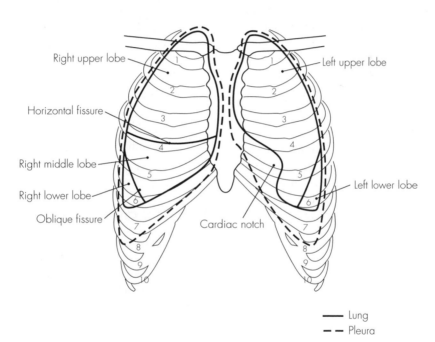

Right upper lobe

Horizontal fissure

Right middle lobe

Right lower lobe

Oblique fissure

Left upper lobe

Left lower lobe

Cardiac notch

—— Lung
- - Pleura

**Fig 7.1**
The pleura and lungs

# 8 The lungs

## DESCRIPTION

The lungs are enclosed within the pleural sacs and separated by the mediastinal structures. Each lung has an apex, base, hilum, three surfaces and three borders.

## RELATIONS

Apex – extends into the root of the neck. The suprapleural membrane and pleural cupola are superior and the subclavian artery leaves a groove on the mediastinal surface of the lung

Base – concave in shape. The right lung is more concave (a higher diaphragm on the right due to the liver's position)

Hilum – structures enter and leave the lung. It is formed mainly by the bronchi, pulmonary arteries, pulmonary veins, bronchial arteries and veins, nerve plexuses, and lymph nodes:

- On the right – superior vena cava and right atrium lie anterior to the hilum, and the azygos vein arches over it
- On the left – thoracic aorta is posterior to the hilum; the aortic arch is superior
- On both sides – phrenic nerve, anterior nerve plexuses and minor vessels lie anteriorly, the vagus nerves and posterior nerve plexuses lie posteriorly

## STRUCTURE

1. Lungs are divided into lobes – three on the right and two on the left. Each lobe is subdivided into triangular bronchopulmonary segments that correspond to the individual segmental bronchi (see above).

2. Right lung has two fissures:
   - Oblique – separates the middle and lower lobes (follows the line from the second vertebral spine to the sixth costochondral junction)
   - Horizontal (transverse) – separates the upper and middle lobes (follows the line from the fourth costochondral junction to join the oblique fissure in the axillary line)

3. Left lung has only one fissure – oblique fissure separating the upper and lower lobes

## POINTS OF INTEREST

- Bronchoscopic anatomy – trachea appears as a glistening tube structure with a red mucosa and regular concentric white tracheal rings. The carina is seen as a sharp ridge and lies slightly to the left of the midline:
  - Right main bronchus is wider and easier to enter:
    Upper lobe bronchus – 2.5 cm from the carina (three o'clock position)
    Middle lobe bronchus – 4.5 cm from the carina (12 o'clock)
    Lower lobe bronchus – 4.5 cm (six o'clock)
  - Left main bronchus is longer (at 5 cm) and narrower:
    Upper lobe bronchus – 5 cm (nine o'clock) with lingular branch centrally at 5.5 cm
    Lower lobe bronchus – 6 cm (six o'clock)

## VASCULAR SUPPLY

1. Pulmonary artery – provides a capillary network for the exchange of the respiratory gases. The pulmonary artery and divisions are concerned solely with alveolar gas exchange and closely follow the bronchial tree divisions. The capillaries in turn feed into the pulmonary veins, which tend to run between the lung segments. The two main pulmonary veins drain separately into the left atrium
2. Bronchial arteries – provide the blood supply to the lungs, bronchi, pleura and lymph nodes. They supply the actual stroma of the lung. There are usually three (variable): one for the right lung and two for the left. They originate from the descending aorta (on the left) and variably from the aorta, an intercostal, internal thoracic or right subclavian artery (on the right). There are two bronchial veins on each side draining into the azygos (right) or hemi-azygos (left) veins. Together with the Thebesian veins of the heart, the bronchial blood flow makes up the 'physiological shunt'

## NERVE SUPPLY

- Tracheobronchial tree and lung:
  - Sensory – vagus (X), recurrent laryngeal
  - Motor – vagus (X) (bronchoconstriction) and sympathetic fibres from T2 to T4 (bronchodilation and minor vasoconstriction)
- Pleura:
  - Parietal sensory – phrenic and intercostal nerves
  - Visceral sensory – autonomic supply

## LYMPHATIC DRAINAGE

1. Superficial plexus drains visceral pleura
2. Deep plexus drains bronchi (as far as alveolar ducts)

Both drain into the bronchopulmonary lymph nodes – then into the tracheobronchial nodes – then into the right and left bronchomediastinal trunks. Variable termination – either directly into great veins of neck, or into thoracic duct (left) and right lymph duct (right).

# 9 The diaphragm

## DESCRIPTION

The diaphragm separates the thoracic and abdominal cavities and is the main muscle of respiration. It consists of a central tendinous portion and a peripheral muscular area. It is dome-shaped in structure and reaches a higher level on the right (fifth rib) than on the left (fifth intercostal space) during end-expiration.

## RELATIONS

Central trefoil tendon – blends with the fibrous pericardium above
Muscle – has a complex origin:
- Costal origin – from the tips of the last six costal cartilages
- Xiphoid origin – from the two small attachments to the posterior surface
- Arcuate ligaments (three):
  - Medial – psoas fascial thickening
  - Lateral – quadratus lumborum fascial thickening
  - Median – fibrous arch between two crura
- Crura:
  - Left – from the first and second lumbar vertebral bodies
  - Right – from the first, second and third lumbar vertebral bodies

## POINTS OF INTEREST

- Three major openings allow for the passage of structures between the thorax and abdomen:
  - At T8 – inferior vena cava (sometimes right phrenic nerve)
  - At T10 – oesophagus, vagi, and left gastric artery and vein
  - At T12 – aorta, thoracic duct and azygos vein
- Further openings transmit:
  - Superior epigastric vessels – between the costal and xiphoid origins
  - Lymphatic vessels – between the costal and xiphoid origins
  - Sympathetic trunk – behind the medial arcuate ligament
  - Right phrenic nerve – pierces the central tendon close to the inferior vena caval opening
  - Left phrenic nerve – pierces muscle just lateral to the pericardial attachment
- Respiration:
  - Diaphragm – moves downwards during inspiration and thus enlarges the thoracic cavity. On expiration it relaxes (and the elastic recoil of the chest wall causes expiration). During quiet breathing the diaphragm is the dominant functioning muscle on inspiration
  - Intercostal muscles – also known to contract on inspiration. This approximates the ribs, and elevates and everts the rib cage increasing the intrathoracic volume. Contraction is also seen on forced expiration (this is presumed to aid rib fixation)
  - Scalene muscles – play a role in inspiration, especially when respiration is deeper. They elevate

the first rib and sternum. In forced inspiration, the erector spinae and pectoral muscles also assist
- Forced expiration – strong contraction of the abdominal and latissimus dorsi muscles pushes the diaphragm upwards

## NERVE SUPPLY

- Motor – phrenic nerve (C3–5)
- Sensory – phrenic nerve to the central tendon, lower thoracic nerves to the muscular regions

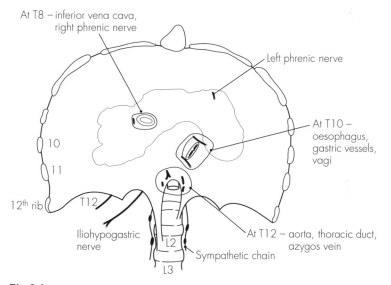

At T8 – inferior vena cava, right phrenic nerve

Left phrenic nerve

At T10 – oesophagus, gastric vessels, vagi

10

11

12<sup>th</sup> rib    T12

Iliohypogastric nerve

L2

L3

Sympathetic chain

At T12 – aorta, thoracic duct, azygos vein

**Fig 9.1**
The diaphragm

# Sample questions – respiratory system

1. Outline your technique for percutaneous tracheostomy with particular reference to the anatomy involved. List the possible complications of this procedure.
2. Draw a simple diagram of the view of the larynx at direct laryngoscopy.
3. What are the effects of damage to the nerve supply of the larynx?
4. Make a simple drawing, with labels, to show the trachea and the main and segmental bronchi.
5. How may the airway be anaesthetised for awake fibreoptic intubation?
6. How may nerve blockade be used to provide pain relief following chest wall trauma?
7. Describe the view seen during bronchoscopic examination.
8. Give a brief account, with a simple diagram, of the anatomy of the diaphragm.

# Cardiovascular System

# 10    The heart

## DESCRIPTION

The heart is a four-chambered, conical, muscular pump in the middle mediastinum. Its borders are:

Right border – right atrium
Left border – left auricular appendage and left ventricle
Anterior surface – right ventricle predominantly
Diaphragmatic surface – right and left ventricles (right atrium)
Posterior surface – left atrium (right atrium)

The surface markings follow a quadrilateral shape (distances from midline): third right costal cartilage (2 cm), second left costal cartilage (3 cm), fifth left intercostal space (7 cm) and sixth right costal cartilage (2 cm).

## STRUCTURE

The heart consists of four chambers:

1. Right atrium – receives deoxygenated blood from the body via the venae cavae (inferior and superior). The outflow of blood occurs through the tricuspid valve into the right ventricle. The sino-atrial node is situated in the upper part of the right atrium, and the atrioventricular node lies near the base of the tricuspid valve
2. Right ventricle – receives blood from the right atrium and expels it through the pulmonary valve and trunk. Some of the rough internal wall

muscle fibres (trabeculae) specialise into papillary muscles, which attach to the tricuspid valve cusps (in a similar fashion to the mitral valve on the left side of the heart). The pulmonary valve is tricuspid and leads into the pulmonary trunk
3. Left atrium – receives oxygenated blood from the lungs via the four pulmonary veins, which open superoposteriorly. The blood then passes through the mitral (bicuspid) valve into the left ventricle
4. Left ventricle – thickest-walled chamber that distributes blood to the body via the aorta. The aortic valve is tricuspid – with right, left and posterior cusps. Small sinuses lie above the cusps that give rise to the two coronary arteries – right and left respectively

## POINTS OF INTEREST

- Conducting system:
  - Sino-atrial node – in the superior right atrial wall (near the superior vena caval opening) and initiates conduction impulse. The node is in direct contact with the atrial cells and causes a wave of depolarisation, resulting in contraction of both atria
  - Atrioventricular node – at the base of the right atrial septal wall (near the tricuspid valve) and receives impulses from the atrial depolarisation. There is no direct neural route between the two nodes, which allows for a slight

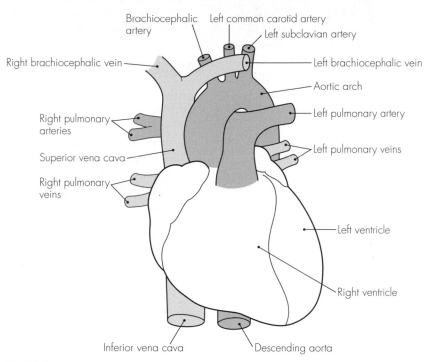

Brachiocephalic artery
Left common carotid artery
Left subclavian artery
Right brachiocephalic vein
Left brachiocephalic vein
Aortic arch
Right pulmonary arteries
Left pulmonary artery
Superior vena cava
Left pulmonary veins
Right pulmonary veins
Left ventricle
Right ventricle
Inferior vena cava
Descending aorta

**Fig 10.1**
The heart

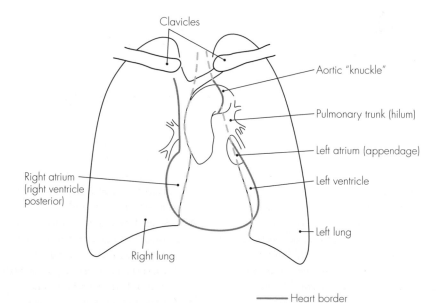

Clavicles
Aortic "knuckle"
Pulmonary trunk (hilum)
Left atrium (appendage)
Right atrium (right ventricle posterior)
Left ventricle
Left lung
Right lung

——— Heart border
– – – "X-ray" shadow

**Fig 10.2**
The heart on chest radiograph

delay and prevents simultaneous atrial and ventricular contraction

- Bundle of His – nerve fibre bundle (AV bundle) that receives the electrical impulse from the AV node and continues within the interventricular septum. At the base it divides into two terminal bundle branches (right and left). These continue in the walls of their respective ventricles, terminating in Purkinje fibres, which penetrate the muscular walls and initiate ventricular contraction
- Pericardium:
  - Heart is enveloped within a conical fibroserous sac – the pericardium. The outer layer is attached to the following structures:
    Adventitia of the great vessels
    Sternopericardial ligament – to the posterior sternum
    Central tendon of diaphragm – where it is fused inferiorly
  - Outer fibrous layer is a tough fibrous structure with openings to allow the aorta, pulmonary trunk and superior vena cava to pass through
  - Serous pericardium has two components:
    Outer parietal pericardium – lines the inner surface of the fibrous sac and becomes continuous with the visceral layer around the great vessels
    Inner visceral pericardium – in direct contact with the heart and forms a potential space between the pericardial layers
  - During embryological folding, sinuses develop in the pericardium:
    Transverse sinus (superiorly) – behind the aorta/pulmonary trunk and in front of superior vena cava
    Oblique sinus (inferiorly) – behind the left atrium (bordered by the inferior vena cava and pulmonary veins)

# VASCULAR SUPPLY

1. Arterial:
   - Right coronary artery – from the right aortic sinus (previously anterior) and descends between the pulmonary trunk and right atrium to run in the anterior atrioventricular groove. Inferiorly, it anastomoses with the left coronary (circumflex) at the inferior interventricular groove. In addition to small atrial and ventricular branches, it gives off two main branches:
   - Right marginal branch – lower border of the heart
   - Posterior interventricular branch – anastomoses with the anterior interventricular branch of the left coronary

   The right coronary artery supplies:
   - Right atrium
   - Part of the left atrium
   - Right ventricle
   - Posterior interventricular septum
   - Sino-atrial node (in 60%)
   - Atrioventricular node (in 80%)

2. Left coronary artery – from the left aortic sinus (previously left posterior) and it lies behind and then lateral to the pulmonary trunk. It also gives off small atrial and ventricular branches, and divides immediately into two main branches:
   - Circumflex artery – runs laterally around the left atrioventricular groove (anastomoses with right coronary as above). This also gives off the left marginal branch
   - Anterior interventricular artery (formerly left anterior descending) – runs down the anterior interventricular groove to anastomose with the posterior

interventricular (from right coronary) as above

The left coronary artery supplies:
- Left atrium
- Left ventricle
- Anterior interventricular septum
- Sino-atrial node (in 40%)
- Atrioventricular node (in 20%)

3. Venous:
- Two-thirds of the drainage is by veins accompanying the arteries – either directly into the right atrium via the anterior cardiac vein, or via the coronary sinus (large venous dilatation posteriorly) into the right atrium. Four veins lead into the coronary sinus:
  - Great cardiac
  - Middle cardiac
  - Small cardiac
  - Oblique
- One-third of the drainage is by small veins, the venae cordis minimae, directly into the cardiac cavity

## NERVE SUPPLY

- Autonomic supply:
  - Parasympathetic – from the vagus nerve (cardio-inhibitory)
  - Sympathetic – cervical (C1–4, C5 and C6, C7–T1) and upper thoracic (T2–5) ganglia (cardio-accelerator) via the superficial and deep cardiac plexuses
- Phrenic nerve (C3–5) supplies the pericardium

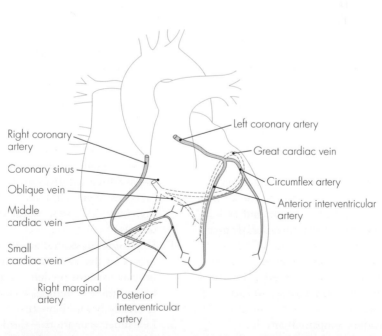

**Fig 10.3**
Blood supply of the heart

# 11    The great vessels

## AORTA

Commences at the aortic valve and terminates at its bifurcation into the common iliac arteries (L4 level). There are four parts:

1.  Ascending – 5 cm long, posterior to sternum. It gives off:
    *   Right coronary artery
    *   Left coronary artery
2.  Arch – runs upwards, backwards and to the left. It gives off:
    *   Brachiocephalic, which divides into:
        *   Right common carotid
        *   Right subclavian
    *   Left common carotid
    *   Left subclavian
    *   Thyroidea ima (occasionally)
3.  Descending thoracic aorta – starts at level T4 and runs down to the aortic opening in the diaphragm (T12). It gives off:
    *   Visceral branches – pericardial, bronchial, oesophageal, mediastinal and phrenic
    *   Somatic branches – posterior intercostals, dorsal, muscular, lateral cutaneous and mammary
4.  Abdominal aorta – starts at the aortic opening in the diaphragm and ends at the common iliac bifurcation. It gives off:
    *   Lumbar arteries (paired)
    *   Visceral arteries (paired) – inferior phrenic, suprarenal, renal and gonadal
    *   Midline (unpaired) arteries:
        *   Celiac trunk – supplies the foregut (via left gastric, common hepatic and splenic)
    *   Superior mesenteric – supplies the midgut (via inferior pancreaticoduodenal, jejunal, ileal, ileocolic, right and middle colic)
    *   Inferior mesenteric – supplies the hindgut (via left colic, sigmoid and superior rectal)

## GREAT ARTERIES OF THE NECK

1.  Brachiocephalic artery – first and largest branch of the aortic arch. It usually gives off no branches and divides into the right common carotid and right subclavian behind the right sternoclavicular joint
2.  Right common carotid artery – ascends within the carotid sheath to divide (opposite the upper border of the thyroid cartilage, C4) into the internal and external carotid arteries
3.  Right subclavian artery – runs (over the cervical pleura and lung apex) to the lateral border of the first rib (grooved) where it becomes the right axillary artery. It gives off five branches: vertebral, internal thoracic, thyrocervical, costocervical and dorsal scapular
4.  Left common carotid artery – second branch of the aortic arch and ascends initially towards the left and then behind the left sternoclavicular joint. It usually has no branches
5.  Left subclavian artery – third branch of the aortic arch, and as on the right side, it grooves the first rib

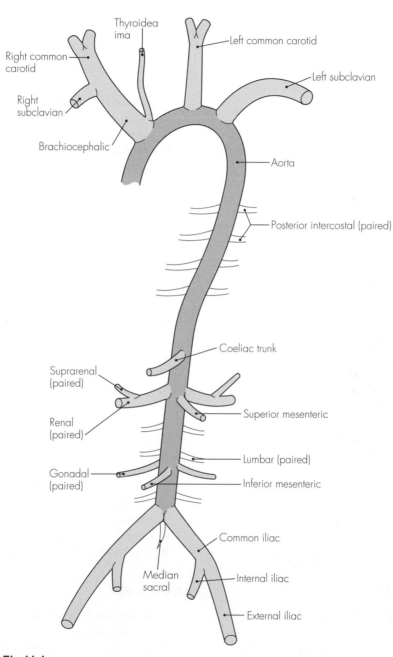

**Fig 11.1**
The aorta and major arterial branches

posteriorly before terminating at its lateral border to become the left axillary artery. It also has five branches (see above)

6. External carotid artery – main blood supply to the head and neck and gives off six branches before bifurcating within the parotid gland:
   - Superior thyroid
   - Ascending pharyngeal
   - Lingual
   - Facial
   - Occipital
   - Posterior auricular
   - Superficial temporal (terminal branch)
   - Maxillary (terminal branch)

7. Internal carotid artery – main blood supply to the intracranial contents and lies initially posterior and lateral to the external carotid (before becoming medial at C2), shortly after which it enters the skull through the carotid canal. There are no cervical branches, but there are 10 branches within the skull:
   - Caroticotympanic and pterygoid (within petrous area)
   - Cavernous, hypophyseal and meningeal (within cavernous area)
   - Ophthalmic
   - Anterior cerebral
   - Middle cerebral
   - Posterior communicating
   - Anterior choroidal

## ARTERIES OF THE LIMBS

### Upper limb

1. Axillary artery – continuation of the subclavian artery and proceeds to become the brachial artery at the lower border of teres major. It gives off:
   - Superior thoracic
   - Thoraco-acromial
   - Lateral thoracic
   - Subscapular
   - Circumflex humeral (anterior and posterior)

2. Brachial artery – extends from the teres major to the lower margins of the antecubital fossa, bifurcating into the radial and ulnar arteries. The branches are:
   - Profunda brachii
   - Ulnar collateral (superior and inferior)
   - Nutrient to humerus

3. Radial artery – lies on the radius along the medial border of the brachioradialis, and it enters to the lateral aspect of the wrist (going through anatomical snuffbox) to terminate in the deep palmar arch. The branches are:
   - Radial recurrent
   - Muscular
   - Carpal
   - Metacarpal
   - Superficial and deep palmar arch

4. Ulnar artery – accompanies the ulnar nerve and lies on the flexor digitorum profundus (lateral to ulnar nerve) before entering the wrist (superficial to flexor retinaculum) and terminating in the superficial palmar arch. The branches are:
   - Ulnar recurrent
   - Common interosseous (divides into anterior and posterior)
   - Muscular
   - Carpal
   - Superficial and deep palmar arch

### Lower limb

1. Common iliac – from the aortic bifurcation at L4

2. External iliac – main continuation of the common iliac and travels down, anteriorly and laterally, deep to the mid-inguinal point and becomes the femoral artery in the thigh. The branches are:

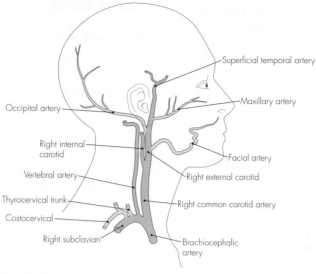

**Fig 11.2**
Major arteries of the head and neck

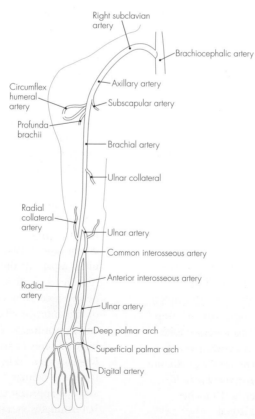

**Fig 11.3**
Arteries of upper limb

- Inferior epigastric – pubic and cremasteric branches
- Deep circumflex iliac

3. Internal iliac – bifurcates into two terminal trunks (anterior and posterior) after running down and posteriorly to end opposite the greater sciatic notch. Multiple branches supply the pelvic organs, genitalia, body wall and lower limb (anterior trunk), and gluteal muscles (posterior trunk)

4. Femoral artery – passes laterally to the femoral vein in the femoral triangle (and medial to the femoral nerve) and descends to enter the popliteal fossa through the adductor hiatus. The branches are:
   - Superficial epigastric
   - Superficial circumflex iliac
   - External pudendal (superficial and deep)
   - Profunda femoris – with perforating arterial branches
   - Descending genicular branch

5. Popliteal artery – continuation of the femoral artery from the adductor magnus above to the popliteus below where it divides into the anterior and posterior tibial arteries

6. Anterior tibial – lies on the anterior surface of the interosseous membrane and enters the ankle (deep to the extensor retinaculum) midway between the malleoli, before becoming the dorsalis pedis artery. Branches supply the knee, anterior compartment, ankle and foot

7. Posterior tibial – descends through the posterior leg compartment deep to the gastrocnemius together with the tibial nerve, and terminates after passing between the medial malleolus and calcaneus in the medial and lateral plantar arteries. Branches supply the fibula, lateral compartment, posterior compartment and foot

## MAJOR VEINS

### Head and neck

1. External jugular vein – drains the scalp and face. It is formed from the posterior division of the retromandibular vein and posterior auricular vein. It runs from the angle of the mandible to the midpoint of the clavicle and then enters the subclavian vein

2. Internal jugular vein – continuation of the sigmoid sinus and runs from the jugular foramen and within the carotid sheath to join with the subclavian vein (behind the sternal end of the clavicle) forming the brachiocephalic vein. It receives numerous tributaries within the neck, including the facial vein, which itself receives the anterior division of the retromandibular vein

### Upper limb

1. Cephalic vein – originates from the dorsal network of hand veins and runs on the radial aspect of the forearm. It receives a median cubital branch before entering the anterior elbow area and ascends lateral to biceps brachii before terminating in the axillary vein

2. Basilic vein – also originates from the dorsal vein network, but runs on the ulnar aspect of the forearm. It also receives a median cubital branch before ascending on the medial aspect of the anterior elbow and forearm, and continues as the axillary vein beyond teres major

3. Median vein of forearm – originates from the palmar venous network and ascends approximately in the midline. It terminates variably in the basilic or median cubital vein

4. Axillary vein – starts at the teres

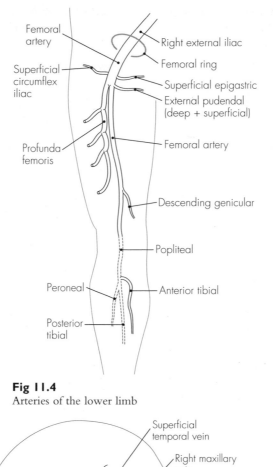
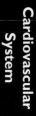

**Fig 11.4**
Arteries of the lower limb

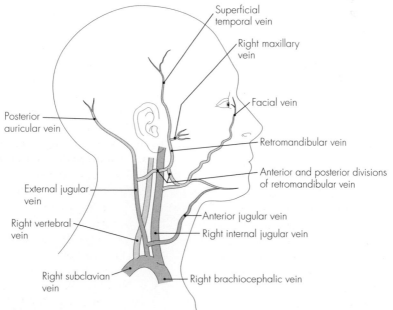

**Fig 11.5**
Major veins of head and neck

major and ends opposite the first rib to continue as the subclavian vein

inferior vena cava (drains blood from below diaphragm)

## Thorax

1. Brachiocephalic vein (bilateral venous, unilateral arterial) – formed from the junction of the internal jugular and subclavian veins behind the sternal clavicle. The longer left and shorter right brachiocephalic veins join behind the first costal cartilage to become the superior vena cava (drains blood from above diaphragm)

## Abdomen

1. External iliac – continuation of the femoral vein (draining the leg) and is joined by the internal iliac (draining the pelvis) to form the common iliac vein in front of the sacroiliac joint
2. Common iliac – left and right ascend and unite at the L5 level to form the

## Lower limb

1. Great saphenous vein – from the medial aspect of the foot and in front of the medial malleolus. It ascends on the medial side to the knee and up to the thigh where it enters the saphenous foramen and joins the femoral vein
2. Small saphenous vein – from the lateral aspect of the foot and behind the lateral malleolus. It ascends in the midline posteriorly and joins the popliteal vein after running between the two heads of the gastrocnemius
3. Posterior tibial vein – runs with the posterior tibial artery and unites with the anterior tibial vein to form the popliteal vein
4. Femoral vein – continuation of the popliteal vein as it emerges from the adductor canal and enters the femoral triangle

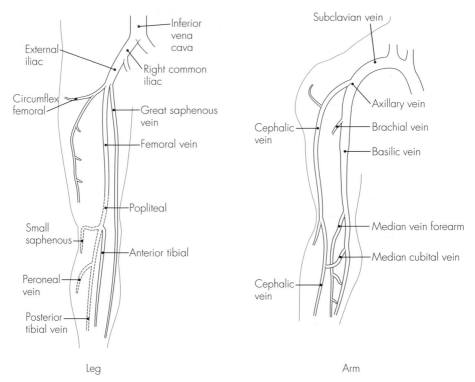

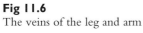

Leg

Arm

**Fig 11.6**
The veins of the leg and arm

# 12    Fetal circulation

- Umbilical vein – oxygenated blood enters the body via the umbilical vein. After mixing with deoxygenated blood in the ductus venosus, it reaches the right atrium (via inferior vena cava that receives blood from trunk and limbs)
- Right atrium – anatomical relationship of the venae cavae ensures that most of the blood in the right atrium (from the inferior vena cava) bypasses the right ventricle and goes directly to the left atrium via the patent foramen ovale
- Left atrium – blood from the left atrium mixes with (deoxygenated) blood from the lungs and is expelled via the left ventricle into the aorta, and ultimately around the body
- Mixing – some blood does not flow directly from the right into the left atrium, but instead it is directed to the right ventricle (mainly blood from the superior vena cava). This deoxygenated blood flows through the lungs and pulmonary trunk, and then via the ductus arteriosus into the aorta
- Transitional circulation – following the clamping of the umbilical cord at birth, and with the large decrease in pulmonary vessel pressure with inspiration, significant pressure and flow changes occur. The fall in right atrial pressure and increase in left atrial pressure causes the foramen ovale to close, as the septum secundum and septum primum oppose. This is an immediate functional closure only. As a result, all blood from the right atrium is now forced into the right ventricle. The ductus arteriosus also constricts due to the high partial pressure of oxygen (functionally complete by 12 hours). The change to adult circulation is complete by 3 months, by which time the foramen ovale is anatomically fused (fossa ovalis) and the ductus arteriosus is obliterated

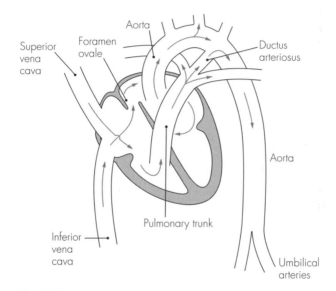

Superior
vena
cava

Foramen
ovale

Aorta

Ductus
arteriosus

Aorta

Pulmonary trunk

Inferior
vena
cava

Umbilical
arteries

**Fig 12.1**
The fetal circulation

# Sample questions – cardiovascular system

1. Describe, with the aid of a simple diagram, the blood supply of the heart. Briefly indicate the areas of myocardium supplied by the coronary arteries and their main branches.
2. Give an account of the arterial supply of the upper limb. List the complications of intra-arterial cannula insertion and indicate the precautions required prior to insertion.
3. Describe the venous drainage of the leg.
4. Using a simple diagram, indicate the special features of the fetal circulation and the subsequent changes following birth.

# Nervous System

# 13 The brain

## DESCRIPTION

There are three main parts of the brain:

Forebrain:
- Telencephalon – consists of the two cerebral hemispheres separated by a longitudinal fissure. The cortex of each hemisphere is made up of gyri and sulci and is separated into lobes. Four major lobes are commonly recognised: frontal, parietal, occipital and temporal
- Diencephalon – lies between the cerebral hemispheres and midbrain. It contains the thalamus and the hypothalamus

Midbrain – connects the forebrain to the hindbrain

Hindbrain – consists of the pons, the medulla oblongata (which exits the cranial cavity through the foramen magnum) and the cerebellum

## VASCULAR SUPPLY

1. Arterial – arterial supply to the brain comes from four arteries: the paired internal carotid arteries and the paired vertebral arteries. These form the circle of Willis from which the anterior, middle and posterior cerebral arteries arise
2. Venous – venous drainage of the brain is via the numerous dural venous sinuses, which drain into the internal jugular vein

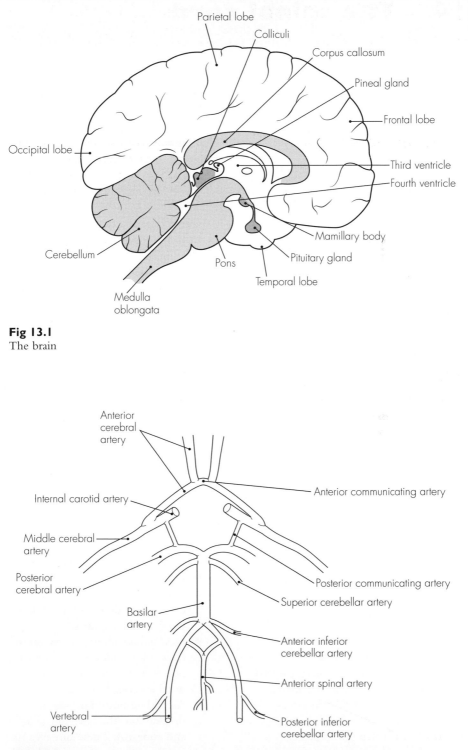

Parietal lobe
Colliculi
Corpus callosum
Pineal gland
Frontal lobe
Third ventricle
Fourth ventricle
Occipital lobe
Mamillary body
Cerebellum
Pons
Pituitary gland
Temporal lobe
Medulla
oblongata

**Fig 13.1**
The brain

Anterior
cerebral
artery
Anterior communicating artery
Internal carotid artery
Middle cerebral
artery
Posterior
cerebral artery
Posterior communicating artery
Basilar
artery
Superior cerebellar artery
Anterior inferior
cerebellar artery
Anterior spinal artery
Vertebral
artery
Posterior inferior
cerebellar artery

**Fig 13.2**
The vascular supply of the brain

# 14    The spinal cord

## DESCRIPTION

The spinal cord is ~45 cm long in the adult and has an approximately cylindrical shape, which is flattened somewhat in the lumbar region. It extends from the cervical area as an extension of the medulla oblongata and continues to the lumbar region, where it terminates in the conus medullaris. A thin thread called the filum terminale continues to attach to the coccyx.

There are normally 31 pairs of spinal nerve roots: eight cervical, 12 thoracic, five lumbar, five sacral and one coccygeal. The elongation of the lumbar and sacral nerve roots, prior to their exit from the intervertebral foramina, forms the cauda equina. There is a wide variation in the relations of the cord throughout the course of life. The spinal cord ends, on average, between L1 and L2 in the adult – and in the newborn it may end at the lower border of L3. However, individual variation between T12 and L3 in the adult is not uncommon.

## STRUCTURE

The spinal cord is roughly circular in cross-section, flattened in the anterior–posterior aspect. There are two major indentations: an anterior median fissure and a posterior median sulcus (which extends further to form the posterior median septum). Further posterolateral sulci exist, along which the posterior nerve roots are seen to exit.

The anterior nerve roots, however, exit without a corresponding groove.

The following structures can be seen on cross-section:

1. Central canal – travels downward from the fourth ventricle. It is continuous throughout the cord and is slightly dilated in the region of the conus medullaris
2. Grey matter – forms the 'H-like' structure in the central regions of the cord. The lateral limbs of grey matter are joined by the transverse commissure. The limbs have an anterior (wider) column or horn and a posterior (narrower) column. The posterior horn has a group of specialised nerve cells, the substantia gelatinosa, at its tip. A lateral grey column can also be seen in the thoracic and upper lumbar area (containing spinal sympathetic cells)
3. White matter – consists of longitudinal nerve fibres divided into the following major tracts:
   - Descending lateral corticospinal tract – major motor tract (fibres cross the midline in the medulla – pyramidal decussation)
   - Descending anterior corticospinal tract – small motor tract (fibres do not decussate until reaching the distal anterior horn cells)
   - Ascending posterior column – divided into the fasciculus gracilis and cuneatus. These subserve fine touch and proprioception (largely uncrossed)

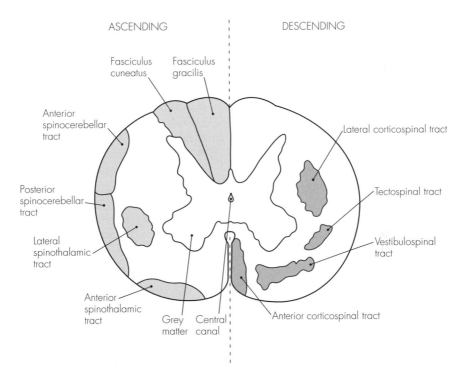

**Fig 14.1**
The spinal cord (transverse section)

- Ascending spinothalamic tracts –
  lateral (pain and temperature –
  cross midline) and anterior/dorsal
  (touch/deep pain – remain
  uncrossed)
- Ascending spinocerebellar tracts –
  anterior and posterior (sensory
  proprioception to the cerebellum)

## VASCULAR SUPPLY

1. Arterial:
   - Anterior spinal artery – formed by
     the union of the vertebral arteries
     at the foramen magnum. It runs
     on the anterior median fissure and
     supplies the larger part of the
     anterior spinal cord
   - Posterior spinal arteries (one or
     two on each side) – formed from
     the posterior cerebellar arteries.
     These are smaller and reinforced
     by spinal branches from a number
     of nearby vessels
   - Radicular arteries also provide
     further blood supply to both the
     anterior and posterior spinal
     arteries. These arise from the
     cervical, thoracic and lumbar
     regions (usually number between
     three and six larger vessels). One
     vessel is often particularly large –
     arteria radicularis magna. It usually
     arises distally and from the left,
     and may provide the dominant
     supply to the lower two-thirds of
     the spinal cord

   Despite the extensive origin, the
   arterial blood supply of the spinal
   cord is vulnerable. The anterior and
   posterior spinal arteries do not have
   direct anastomoses and cord
   infarction is possible after thrombosis,
   hypotension, surgical occlusion,
   trauma, and vasoconstriction.

2. Venous:
   - By a series of venous plexuses or
     channels (anterior, posterior and
     lateral), which in turn drain into
     segmental veins, including the
     vertebral, azygos, lumbar and
     lateral sacral veins

## DESCRIPTION

The central nervous system is covered with three contiguous membranes called the meninges. These protect and support the neural tissue. The three layers are the dura mater (outermost), the arachnoid mater and the pia mater (innermost). The subdural (potential) space separates the dura and arachnoid mater, and the subarachnoid (actual) space separates the arachnoid and pia mater – latter closely applied to the neural tissue.

The spinal meninges are the equivalent of the cranial meninges. The spinal dura is separated from the periosteum by the extradural (epidural) space.

## STRUCTURE

1. Extradural (epidural) space – separates the dura mater from the periosteum. It extends from the foramen magnum to the sacral hiatus. The space is roughly triangular in cross-section, with a small anterior and two larger posterolateral compartments. The space also extends a short distance laterally through the spinal foramina (as the nerve roots exit). The distance from the posterior epidural space border to the dural sac varies from ~6 mm in the lumbar region to only 1 mm in the cervical region. The epidural space is found variably 3–5 cm beneath the skin (range 2–7 cm). The epidural space has the following contents:
   - Fat (semifluid)
   - Lymphatics
   - Arteries
   - Veins (the valveless, vertebral, venous plexuses of Bateson – forming a communication from pelvic to cerebral veins)

2. Dura mater – dense, fibrous tissue as a double layer (the outer layer attaches at foramen magnum [and to C2 and C3], the inner layer is the continuation of the cerebral dura). The dura extends as far as the second sacral segment (variably L5–S3). It also ensheathes the filum terminale (an extension of pia mater), which attaches to the coccygeal periosteum. The dura is attached anteriorly by slips to the posterior longitudinal ligament and laterally to prolongations around the nerve roots, but it remains free posteriorly

3. Subdural space – a potential space as the arachnoid mater is closely applied to the dura (with a thin film of serous fluid in between)

4. Arachnoid mater – thin, delicate membrane lining dural sheath (and has similar small extensions along nerve roots)

5. Subarachnoid (spinal) space – actual space containing cerebrospinal fluid (CSF)

6. Pia mater – vascular connective sheath that closely invests the spinal cord. It is thickened anteriorly (linea splendens) and has lateral strands for attachments to the dura (ligamentum denticulatum). Posteriorly it attaches to the dura by an incomplete sheet of pia (posterior subarachnoid septum). The inferior attachment of the pia

mater to the coccyx is via its continuation – filum terminale

# POINTS OF INTEREST

- Cerebrospinal fluid (CSF):
  - Volume – ~150 ml (roughly equal to daily production), only 25 ml of which is contained in the spinal/subarachnoid space
  - Production – by the choroid plexuses of the lateral, third and fourth ventricles. It passes from the lateral ventricles to the third ventricle via the paired interventricular foramina (of Munro), and then via the cerebral aqueduct to the fourth ventricle. The CSF then flows from the fourth ventricle to the subarachnoid spinal space through the paired lateral foramina of Lushka and the median foramen of Magendie
  - Absorption – ~80% is absorbed via the arachnoid villi (projections of arachnoid mater) in the cerebral venous sinuses. The remaining 20% is absorbed by spinal arachnoid villi or by lymphatic drainage. The CSF pressure is gravity-dependent and ranges from 6 to 10 cm (of CSF) when lying, to subatmospheric cervically and 20–40 cm in the lumbar area when sitting
  - Composition – is approximately:
    Osmolality = 280 mOsm
    Specific gravity = 1005
    pH 7.4
    Glucose = 1.5–4.0 mmol $l^{-1}$
    Sodium = 140–150 mmol $l^{-1}$
    Chloride = 120–130 mmol $l^{-1}$
    Bicarbonate = 25–30 mmol $l^{-1}$
    Protein = 0.15–0.3 g $l^{-1}$
    Cells = less than five lymphs $mm^{-3}$

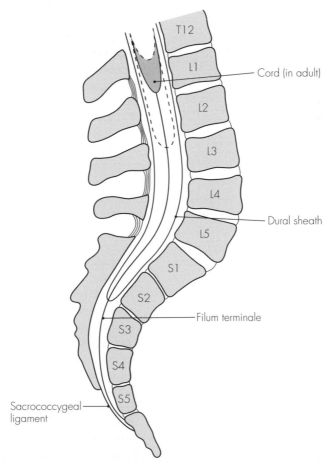

Cord (in adult)

Dural sheath

Filum terminale

Sacrococcygeal
ligament

**Fig 15.1**
The termination of the spinal cord

# 16　The spinal nerves

## DESCRIPTION

These number 31 pairs in total: eight cervical, 12 thoracic, five lumbar, five sacral and one coccygeal. The nerves are mixed (i.e. contain sensory and motor fibres) and are formed from the fusion of ventral (anterior) motor and dorsal (posterior) sensory roots. Unlike the ventral roots, the dorsal sensory roots contain a ganglion located just prior to the fusion of the roots.

The spinal nerves exit from the vertebral canal through the intervertebral foramina, and the nerve roots are sheathed in meningeal membranes – dura extending as far as the fusion to form the spinal nerve.

Once fused, the spinal nerves immediately give off a small meningeal branch (which supplies the vertebral structures) and then divide into two major nerves: the dorsal and ventral rami. There is also a branch that links to the sympathetic ganglionic chain – these are called the rami communicantes.

## STRUCTURE

1.  Dorsal (posterior) primary rami – generally smaller than the ventral rami and divide into medial and lateral branches. They are concerned with the innervation of the back (skin and muscles). The innervation is characteristically segmental or dermatomal in distribution. A few dorsal rami are exceptional:
    * First cervical dorsal ramus is entirely motor, larger and does not have medial and lateral branches. It supplies the muscles of the suboccipital triangle
    * Second cervical dorsal ramus is also large and divides into a large medial branch (which becomes the greater occipital nerve) and a smaller lateral (motor) branch
    * Coccygeal dorsal ramus is very small, undivided and supplies the skin over the coccyx
2.  Ventral (anterior) primary rami – generally larger, these supply the arm, leg and the anterior/lateral aspects of the torso. Some ventral rami unite and form nerve plexuses: cervical, brachial and lumbosacral. These are discussed below. The thoracic ventral rami remain, however, independent of each other, separated by the ribs. They, like the dorsal rami, innervate segmentally (dermatomal distribution)

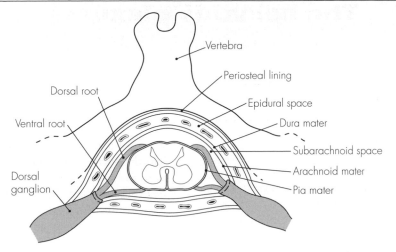

**Fig 16.1**
The spinal meninges

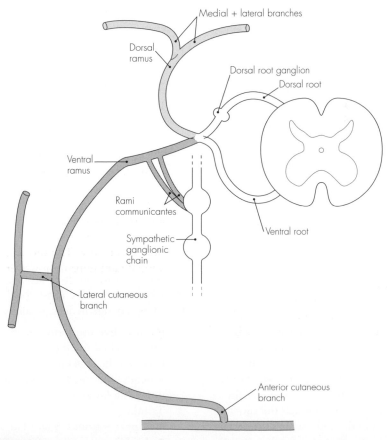

**Fig 16.2**
The distribution of the spinal nerve

# 17    The nervous plexuses

## DESCRIPTION

The ventral rami of the spinal nerves unite and form complex plexuses in the cervical, brachial, lumbar and sacrococcygeal regions. These supply the neck, arms and legs respectively.

## CERVICAL PLEXUS

This is formed from the ventral rami of C1–4. It is responsible for the innervation of the skin of the head, neck, and the neck and diaphragmatic musculature. The rami (except C1-motor only) divide into ascending and descending branches, which form the three major loops of the plexus. These further divide into deep (motor) and superficial (sensory) branches.

There are four major groups of branches:

1. Communicating branches – pass to the hypoglossal nerve, vagus nerve and cervical sympathetic chain
2. Phrenic nerve – motor nerve to the diaphragm. It also transmits proprioceptive fibres from the diaphragm as well as pleural and pericardial branches. The phrenic nerve is derived from C3 to C5. The three roots unite at the lateral edge of scalenus anterior before descending medially and anteriorly over the muscle. The nerve then crosses over the subclavian artery and under the subclavian vein (through the thoracic inlet). On the right side, the nerve follows the great veins and pierces the central tendon just lateral to the inferior vena caval opening. On the left, the nerve crosses over the aortic arch (in front of the vagus nerve) and over the lung root and pericardium to pierce the diaphragm just lateral to the pericardial attachment
3. Superficial branches – sensory to neck. These can be divided into three groups:
   - Ascending:
     - Lesser occipital nerve – (C2)
     - Great auricular nerve – (C2, C3)
   - Descending – supraclavicular nerves – (C3, C4)
   - Transverse – anterior cutaneous nerve of neck – (C2, C3)
4. Deep branches – motor to neck muscles. These supply the anterior vertebral muscles and send additional small contributions to the scalenus medius, levator scapulae, sternomastoid and trapezius

## BRACHIAL PLEXUS

Formed from the ventral rami of C5–8 and T1. Occasionally, there may be a significant contribution from C4 (prefixed) or from T2 (post-fixed). The following arrangement is usually seen:

1. Roots – five roots emerge from the intervertebral foramina and continue between the scalenus medius and scalenus anterior. Here the roots unite as follows into:
2. Trunks:
   - Upper – from C5 and C6
   - Middle – continues from C7
   - Lower – from C8 and T1

Nervous
System

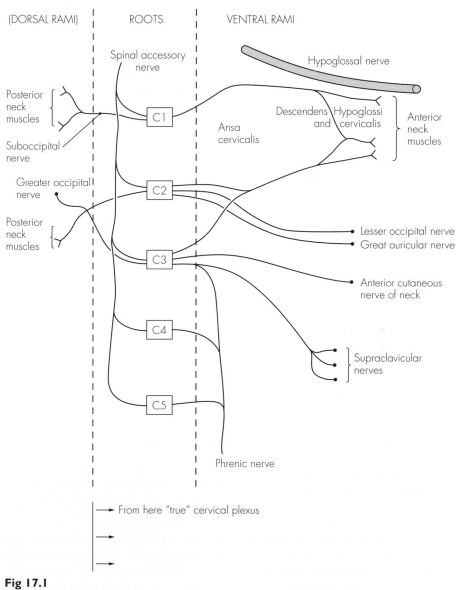

(DORSAL RAMI)    ROOTS    VENTRAL RAMI

Spinal accessory
nerve

Hypoglossal nerve

Posterior
neck
muscles

C1

Descendens Hypoglossi
and cervicalis

Anterior
neck
muscles

Ansa
cervicalis

Suboccipital
nerve

Greater occipital
nerve

C2

Posterior
neck
muscles

Lesser occipital nerve
Great auricular nerve

C3

Anterior cutaneous
nerve of neck

C4

Supraclavicular
nerves

C5

Phrenic nerve

From here "true" cervical plexus

**Fig 17.1**
The cervical plexus

The trunks emerge from between the scalene and pass downward over the posterior neck triangle and first rib. At the lateral border of the first rib the trunks divide into:

3. Divisions – each trunk divides into an anterior and posterior division behind the clavicle. These divisions continue on into the axilla and form into:
4. Cords – according to their position around the axillary artery:
   - Lateral – anterior divisions of upper and middle trunks
   - Medial – anterior division of lower trunk
   - Posterior – posterior divisions of all three trunks

The brachial plexus is surrounded by a sheath of fibrous tissue, from its origin (interscalene sheath) to the axilla. The important larger branches of the brachial plexus are:

1. Supraclavicular branches:
   - Dorsal scapular nerve (C5) – to the rhomboids
   - Long thoracic nerve (C5–7) – to the serratus anterior
   - Small branches to scalenus/longus colli muscles
   - Suprascapular nerve (C5, 6) – to the scapular area
   - Nerve to subclavius (C5, 6) – to the subclavius
2. Infraclavicular branches:
   - Lateral cord:
     - Lateral pectoral nerve (C5–7) – to the pectoralis major and minor
     - Musculocutaneous nerve (C5–7) – to the biceps, brachialis and skin (via the lateral cutaneous nerve of the forearm)
   - Medial cord:
     - Medial pectoral nerve (C8–T1) – to the pectoralis minor

- Medial cutaneous nerve of the arm (C8–T1)
- Medial cutaneous nerve of the forearm (C8–T1)
   - Posterior cord:
     - Upper subscapular nerve (C5, 6) – to the subscapularis
     - Lower subscapular nerve (C5, 6) – to the subscapularis and teres major
     - Thoracodorsal nerve (C5–7) – to the latissimus dorsi
     - Axillary nerve (C5, 6) – to the deltoid
3. Radial nerve (C5–T1) – formed from the posterior cord
4. Median nerve (C6–T1) – formed from the medial and lateral cords
5. Ulnar nerve (C8, T1) – formed from the medial cord

## LUMBAR PLEXUS

Formed from ventral rami of L1–4. There may be a contribution from T12 (in 50%) or from L5. The plexus assembles within psoas major (anterior to the transverse processes of the L2–5). The usual arrangement is:

1. L1 divides into upper and lower divisions. The upper division gives off the iliohypogastric and ilioinguinal nerves. The lower division joins with a branch of L2 to form the genitofemoral nerve
2. L2–4 divide into dorsal and ventral divisions. The dorsal divisions of L2 and L3 form the lateral cutaneous nerve of the thigh and L2–4 form the femoral nerve. The ventral branches join to form the obturator nerve
3. L4 and L5 branches also join to form the lumbosacral trunk, which becomes part of the sacrococcygeal plexus

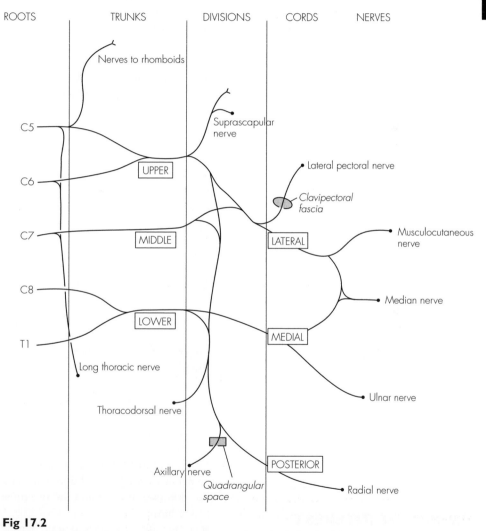

ROOTS        TRUNKS       DIVISIONS     CORDS     NERVES

Nerves to rhomboids

C5

Suprascapular
nerve

UPPER

Lateral pectoral nerve

C6

*Clavipectoral
fascia*

C7

MIDDLE

LATERAL

Musculocutaneous
nerve

C8

Median nerve

LOWER

MEDIAL

T1

Long thoracic nerve

Ulnar nerve

Thoracodorsal nerve

POSTERIOR

Axillary nerve

*Quadrangular
space*

Radial nerve

**Fig 17.2**
The brachial plexus

## SACROCOCCYGEAL PLEXUS

There is a wide variation in constitution. The sacral plexus is formed from L4–5 and S1–4. The coccygeal part is formed from S4, S5 and the coccygeal nerve:

1. L4 and L5 form the lumbosacral trunk at the medial border of psoas major. This travels over the pelvic brim and joins S1
2. Ventral rami of S1–4, with S5 and Co. 1 join the plexus within the pelvis

The sacral plexus has numerous vessels passing in between the nerve trunks. These are the inferior gluteal, superior gluteal, iliolumbar and internal pudendal vessels. The most important nerve branches are:

1. Superior gluteal nerve (L4 and L5, S1)
2. Inferior gluteal nerve (L5, S1 and S2)
3. Posterior femoral cutaneous nerve (S1–3)
4. Perforating cutaneous nerve (S2 and S3)
5. Pudendal nerve (S2–4)
6. Sciatic nerve (S2–4) – largest nerve in the body and supplies (together with the femoral nerve) the lower limb

The coccygeal part of the plexus is small. S4, S5 and Co. 1 join to form the anococcygeal nerve, and this supplies the skin over the coccyx.

## POINTS OF INTEREST

- Regional anaesthetic blockade is possible by injecting a local anaesthetic solution around the nerves of a plexus. Brachial plexus blockade is the most commonly performed major peripheral nerve block, but the cervical and lumbar plexuses may also be targeted

- Brachial plexus block – large number of techniques described, but each falls into one of four groups:
  - Interscalene
  - Supraclavicular
  - Axillary
  - Infraclavicular
- No one technique is demonstrably better than the others, and each has different benefits and complications. The more common complications include pneumothorax, phrenic nerve palsy, stellate ganglion block, recurrent laryngeal nerve palsy, subarachnoid injection and vertebral artery injection. The details of how to perform these blocks are well described in the many excellent texts of regional anaesthesia
- Cervical plexus block – provides good analgesia of the skin of the occipital region, posterior neck and shoulders. The superficial branches of the plexus provide the sensory supply. These are best located by turning the patient's head slightly away from the side to be blocked. The point of needle entry is taken from a line drawn laterally from the cricoid cartilage where it meets the posterior border of the sternomastoid. A needle inserted at this point at right angles to the skin will pop through the cervical fascia, where 10 ml local anaesthetic is then injected
- Lumbar plexus block – provides analgesia to the lower abdominal skin, the skin over the hip and the proximal lower limb:
  - Classically, the original approach was paravertebral. This involved the patient lying prone, and a point 4 cm lateral to the spinal process of L3 used as the entry point. The transverse process is contacted at ~5 cm depth, at which point the needle is directed slightly cephalad and medially, and 'walked off' the

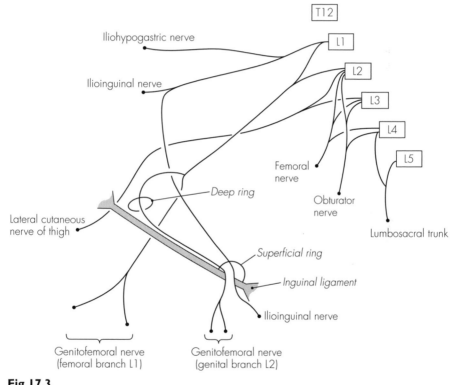

Iliohypogastric nerve

Ilioinguinal nerve

T12

L1

L2

L3

L4

L5

Femoral
nerve

Deep ring

Obturator
nerve

Lateral cutaneous
nerve of thigh

Lumbosacral trunk

Superficial ring

Inguinal ligament

Ilioinguinal nerve

Genitofemoral nerve
(femoral branch L1)

Genitofemoral nerve
(genital branch L2)

**Fig 17.3**
The lumbar plexus

process for a further 2 cm. Solution (30 ml) is then injected

- Direct lumbar plexus block technique is identical, except that the needle is not angled medially, only cephalad, once the transverse process is contacted

- Modified three-in-one technique may also be used. This relies on the spread of the solution within the inguinal canal reaching the lumbar roots, and consequently higher volumes of solution are required

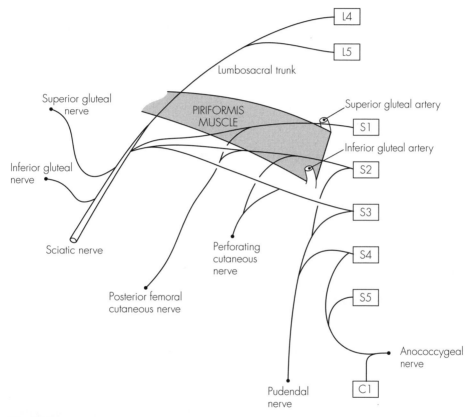

**Fig 17.4**
The sacrococcygeal plexus

# 18  The major peripheral nerves

These are divided into groups according to the area of supply.

## UPPER LIMB

1.  Radial nerve – continuation of the posterior cord of the brachial plexus (C5–T1). It descends posterior to the axillary and brachial arteries and crosses the tendons of latissimus dorsi and teres major. It passes between the long and medial heads of triceps (accompanying profunda brachii vessels) before running posteriorly around the spiral groove of the humerus. It then pierces the lateral intermuscular septum and runs forward between brachioradialis and brachialis muscles. It terminates over the lateral epicondyle in two branches – superficial radial nerve and posterior interosseous nerve. The radial nerve supplies:
    *   Muscular branches to – triceps, anconeus, brachialis, brachioradialis and extensor carpi radialis longus
    *   Cutaneous branches – posterior cutaneous nerve of the arm, posterior cutaneous nerve of the forearm and lower lateral cutaneous nerve of the arm
    *   Posterior interosseous nerve – entirely motor to the extensors of the forearm and hand, and runs through the supinator muscle
    *   Superficial radial nerve – entirely sensory and runs under brachioradialis (with radial artery) before dividing above the wrist

into digital branches. It supplies the dorsal thumb base, radial side of back of hand and the back of the radial three and a half digits

2.  Musculocutaneous nerve – arises from the lateral cord (C5–7). It runs from behind the pectoralis minor (lateral to axillary artery) and descends between the biceps and brachialis. It terminates in the lateral cutaneous nerve of the forearm. It supplies:
    *   Muscular branches to – coracobrachialis, biceps and brachialis
    *   Sensory branches – from the lateral cutaneous nerve of the forearm, supplying the skin over the lateral forearm and wrist

3.  Median nerve – arises from the medial and lateral cords (C6–T1). Initially anterior to the axillary artery, it then runs laterally and crosses the brachial artery at the mid-humerus level to become medial in the antecubital fossa. Running on coracobrachialis and brachialis, it passes under the bicipital aponeurosis and enters the forearm between the flexor digitorum profundus and flexor digitorum superficialis. It emerges laterally at the wrist to run under the flexor retinaculum (in the carpal tunnel) and terminates in two branches (medial and lateral). The median nerve supplies:
    *   Muscular branches to – pronator teres, flexor carpi ulnaris, palmaris longus, flexor digitorum superficialis, three thenar muscles and lateral two lumbricals

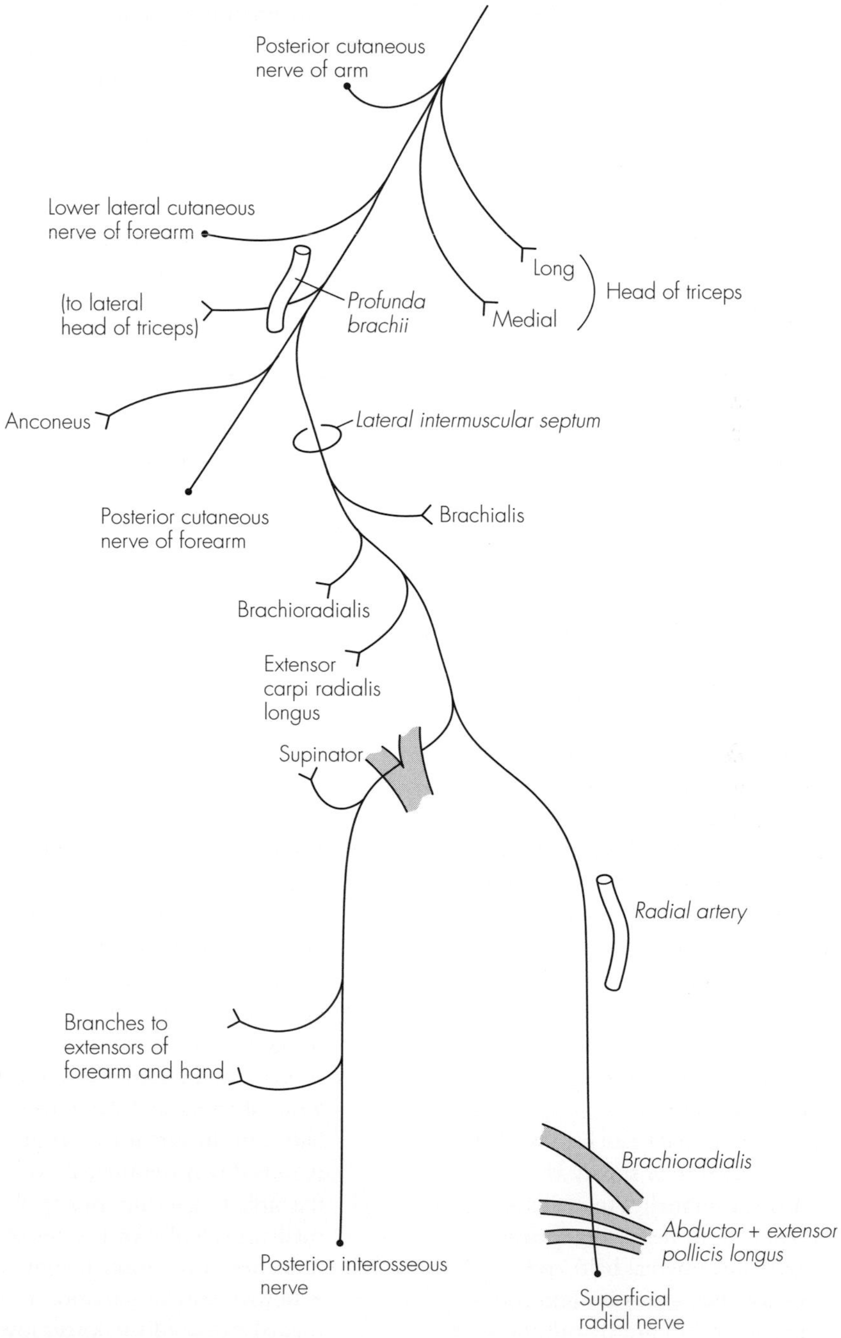

Posterior cutaneous
nerve of arm

Lower lateral cutaneous
nerve of forearm

(to lateral
head of triceps)

*Profunda
brachii*

Long

Medial

Head of triceps

Anconeus

*Lateral intermuscular septum*

Posterior cutaneous
nerve of forearm

Brachialis

Brachioradialis

Extensor
carpi radialis
longus

Supinator

Radial artery

Branches to
extensors of
forearm and hand

*Brachioradialis*

*Abductor + extensor
pollicis longus*

Posterior interosseous
nerve

Superficial
radial nerve

**Fig 18.1**
The radial nerve

- Sensory branches to – thenar eminence and front of radial three and a half digits
- Anterior interosseous branch – given off high up between the heads of the pronator teres, and descends to supply the flexor pollicis longus, flexor digitorum profundus (radial half) and pronator quadratus
- Palmar branch – crosses superficially over the flexor retinaculum and supplies sensation to the ball of thumb and palm of the hand
- Lateral terminal branch gives off a recurrent muscular branch to the abductor pollicis brevis, flexor pollicis brevis and opponens pollicis. The medial branch continues to supply the sensation to the hand and fingers as above

4. Ulnar nerve – originates from the medial cord (C8, T1). It arises medially and continues on coracobrachialis, before passing deep through the medial intermuscular septum. It approximates the medial head of the triceps to run behind the medial epicondyle and enters the forearm between the two heads of the flexor carpi ulnaris. It continues initially deep to the flexor carpi ulnaris and then laterally (on top of the flexor digitorum profundus). It crosses superficially to the flexor retinaculum to terminate (superficial and deep terminal branches) over the pisiform bone. The supply is:
   - Muscular branches to – flexor carpi ulnaris, flexor digitorum profundus (medial half) and intrinsic hand muscles (except lateral two lumbricals and thenar muscles)
   - Sensory branches to – front and back aspects of medial hand and medial one and a half fingers

- Palmar cutaneous branch – arises in the mid-forearm and supplies the hypothenar skin
- Dorsal branch – also arises in the mid-forearm and supplies the ulnar border of the hand
- Terminal branches supply sensation as above (superficial branch) and motor to hypothenar muscles (three), ulnar two lumbricals, interossei and adductor pollicis

## LOWER LIMB

1. Femoral nerve – derived from L2–4 and formed within the psoas major. It descends between the psoas major (laterally) and iliacus, and enters the thigh lateral to the femoral artery and under the inguinal ligament. Within the femoral triangle it splits immediately into its terminal branches, via the anterior and posterior divisions. The femoral nerve supplies:
   - Muscular branches to – pectineus and sartorius (anterior), and quadriceps femoris (posterior)
   - Sensory branches – intermediate cutaneous nerve of thigh and medial cutaneous nerve of thigh (anterior), and the terminal saphenous nerve (posterior)
   - Saphenous nerve – largest branch of the femoral nerve runs initially lateral and then medial over the femoral artery and descends between the sartorius and gracilis. It runs down the medial border of the tibia to pass anterior to the medial malleolus and terminates in branches to the foot. It supplies an extensive area of sensation to the medial aspect of the knee, lower leg, ankle and foot

2. Obturator nerve – derived from L2–4 and continues from its formation within the psoas major along the

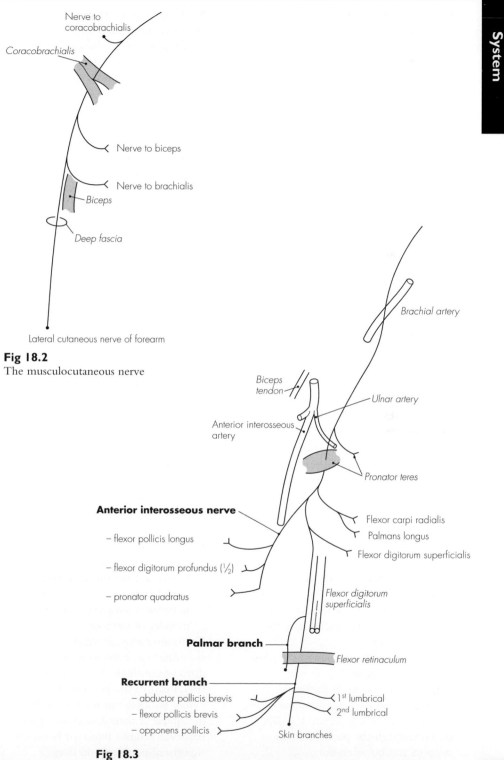

**Fig 18.2**
The musculocutaneous nerve

**Fig 18.3**
The median nerve

pelvic sidewall and posterior to the common iliac vessels. After passing over the pelvic brim, it enters the obturator canal and divides into anterior and posterior divisions. It supplies:

- Muscular branches to – adductor longus and brevis, pectineus and gracilis (anterior), and obturator externus and half adductor magnus (posterior)
- Sensory branches to – hip joint and medial skin over thigh (anterior) and knee joint (posterior)

3. Sciatic nerve – formed from L4 and L5 and S1–3 (on pyriformis) and passes back through the greater sciatic foramen and lies deep to the gluteus maximus. It runs down on the gemellus superior and inferior, and lies initially posterior to the acetabulum. From a point midway between the greater trochanter and ischial tuberosity, it runs directly down on the quadratus femoris and adductor magnus. It passes between the two heads of the biceps femoris and continues in the posterior midline of the thigh. It terminates in the common peroneal and tibial nerves above the knee. The sciatic nerve supplies:

- Muscular branches to – semitendinosus, semimembranosus, adductor magnus (half) and biceps femoris
- Nerve to quadratus femoris – also inferior gemellus and sensory to the hip joint
- Nerve to obturator internus – also superior gemellus

4. Tibial nerve – arises in the lower third of the thigh as the terminal branch of the sciatic nerve. It passes down through the popliteal fossa, deep to and between the semimembranosus and biceps femoris.

It leaves the fossa between the heads of the gastrocnemius to run on the tibialis posterior in the calf, gradually sloping medially. It winds behind the medial malleolus (with the posterior tibial artery medially and flexor hallucis longus tendon laterally) to enter the foot under the flexor retinaculum, and terminates into the medial and lateral plantar nerves. The nerve supplies:

- Muscular branches to – popliteus, gastrocnemius, soleus and plantaris (in popliteal fossa), and tibialis posterior, flexor digitorum longus, flexor hallucis longus and soleus (in the calf and foot)
- Sensory branches to – sural nerve (in popliteal fossa) and medial calcaneal nerve (foot)
- Sural nerve – arises from the popliteal fossa and becomes superficial to run laterally down the lower leg. It passes behind the lateral malleolus to supply sensation to the lateral foot
- Terminal branches supply the foot via the medial and lateral plantar branches. The sensory supply is to the medial two-thirds of the sole of the foot and plantar medial three and a half toes (medial plantar) and lateral one-third of the sole of the foot and plantar lateral one and a half toes (lateral plantar). Together with the branches of the common peroneal nerve they supply the intrinsic muscles of the foot

5. Common peroneal nerve – derived from the sciatic nerve in the lower third of the thigh. It runs in the lateral part of the popliteal fossa before winding around the neck of the fibula. It then divides (deep to peroneus longus) into two branches – superficial peroneal and deep peroneal nerves. It supplies:

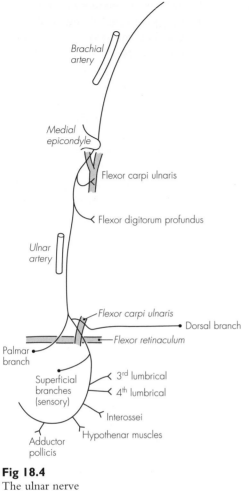

**Fig 18.4**
The ulnar nerve

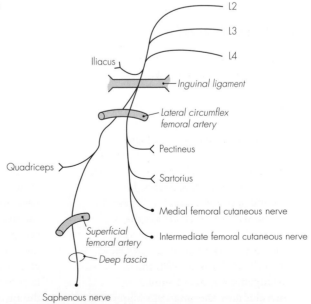

**Fig 18.5**
The femoral nerve

- No muscular branches
- Sensory branches to – sural communicating nerve and lateral cutaneous nerve of the calf
- Superficial peroneal (previously musculocutaneous) nerve – lies over the lateral surface of the fibula and becomes subcutaneous and anterior over the ankle. It supplies muscular branches to the peroneus longus and brevis. It supplies sensation to the lower outer aspect of the lower leg and terminates in sensory branches to the dorsum of the foot
- Deep peroneal (previously anterior tibial) nerve – lies on the interosseous membrane and passes anterior to the tibia at the ankle. Muscular branches pass to the tibialis anterior, extensor digitorum longus, extensor hallucis longus and peroneus tertius. The terminal branches supply the extensor digitorum brevis (lateral) and the web space between first and second toes (medial)

## ABDOMINAL WALL

1. The innervation of the abdominal wall is by the ventral (anterior) primary rami of T7–L1. The segmental (dermatomal) distribution is: the xiphisternum is supplied by T7, the umbilicus by T10 and the groin by L1. The intercostal nerves, T7–11, and the subcostal nerve, T12, maintain a course between the second and third muscular layers. In the thorax, these layers are the internal and innermost intercostal muscles. As the nerve muscles run into the abdominal wall, the arrangement remains similar – muscles now the internal oblique and transversus abdominus.
3. The first lumbar nerve (from the lumbar plexus) divides into the iliohypogastric and ilioinguinal nerves. The course of these nerves differs from the usual pattern. The iliohypogastric nerve pierces the internal oblique, to run deep to the external oblique, and supplies the pubic skin. The ilioinguinal nerve also pierces the internal oblique and runs across the inguinal canal (anterior to the spermatic cord). It exits the canal via the external ring or adjacent aponeurosis, and supplies the scrotum/labium majus and upper thigh.
3. Each nerve from T7 to T12 also gives off a lateral cutaneous branch (with anterior and posterior branches), which divides in the mid-axillary line. These branches supply the skin of the flank and back in the relevant distribution. The iliohypogastric and subcostal nerves, however, do not have a divided lateral cutaneous nerve, but continue down to supply the skin over the upper lateral buttock. The ilioinguinal nerve has no lateral cutaneous branch.

## INTERCOSTAL NERVES

1. These are derived from the ventral (anterior) primary rami of T1–11. After emerging from the intervertebral foramen (and giving off the dorsal primary ramus), the ventral rami have small branches that communicate with the sympathetic ganglia – rami communicantes. At this point, the intercostal nerves lie for a short distance between the pleura and inner muscle layer. The nerves pass posterior and then below the intercostal arteries to run in the layer between the innermost and internal intercostal muscle, and

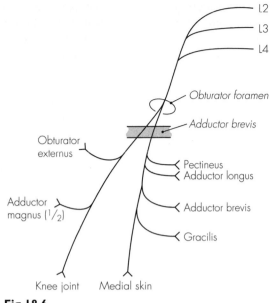

**Fig 18.6**
The obturator nerve

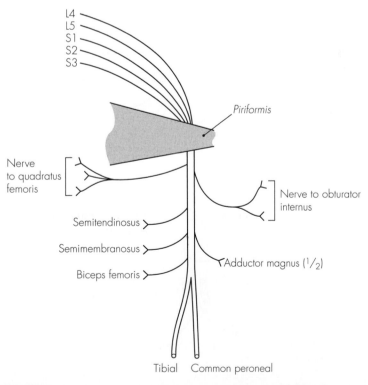

**Fig 18.7**
The sciatic nerve

closely follow the subcostal grooves of the ribs. Typically, there are the following branches:

- Collateral branch – arises at the angle of the rib and supplies the underlying muscle only
- Lateral cutaneous branch – arises at the mid-axillary line and supplies sensation to the overlying skin via anterior and posterior branches
- Anterior cutaneous branch – arises over the anterior chest/abdominal wall to supply sensation to the overlying skin

2. There are some intercostal nerves with atypical features. T1 has no lateral or anterior cutaneous branches, and supplies the lower part of the brachial plexus. T2 has an atypical lateral cutaneous branch, the intercostobrachial nerve, which arches over the axillary roof (supplying the medial upper arm sensation). T7–11 have an abdominal course but maintain their position between the second and third muscular layers.

3. T12 is called the subcostal nerve (runs below the 12th rib), but has similar branches to the typical intercostal nerve.

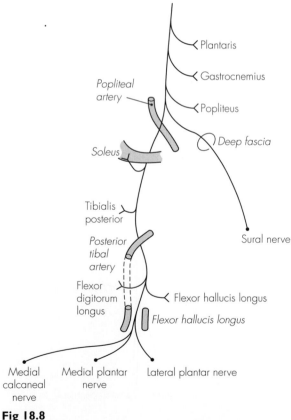

**Fig 18.8**
The tibial nerve

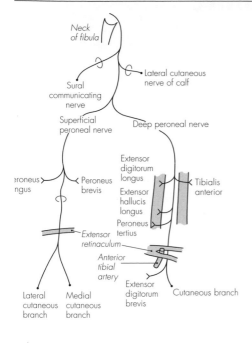

Neck of fibula

Sural communicating nerve

Lateral cutaneous nerve of calf

Superficial peroneal nerve

Deep peroneal nerve

Extensor digitorum longus

Peroneus longus

Peroneus brevis

Tibialis anterior

Extensor hallucis longus

Peroneus tertius

Extensor retinaculum

Anterior tibial artery

Extensor digitorum brevis

Cutaneous branch

Lateral cutaneous branch

Medial cutaneous branch

ise Anatomy
aesthesia

**Fig 18.9**
The common peroneal nerve

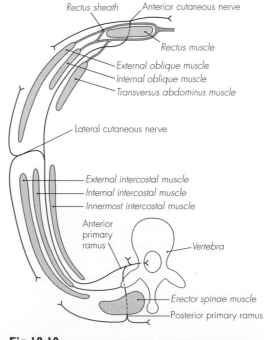

Rectus sheath    Anterior cutaneous nerve

Rectus muscle

External oblique muscle

Internal oblique muscle

Transversus abdominus muscle

Lateral cutaneous nerve

External intercostal muscle

Internal intercostal muscle

Innermost intercostal muscle

Anterior primary ramus

Vertebra

Erector spinae muscle

Posterior primary ramus

**Fig 18.10**
A typical intercostal nerve

# 19 The autonomic nervous system

The autonomic nervous system is divided into two functionally and anatomically different nervous systems: sympathetic and parasympathetic. Characteristically, the autonomic nervous system has myelinated nerves, which emerge from the central nervous system, synapse in a ganglion and are then distributed to the end organ as small non-myelinated fibres.

Anatomically, the sympathetic nervous system has the ganglia close to the outflow from the cord, and this is facilitated by the sympathetic chain of ganglia in close proximity to the vertebral column. The cell bodies of the sympathetic system are found in the lateral horn of the spinal cord, from T1 to L2. The white rami communicantes (preganglionic) relay the impulses from these cell bodies to the sympathetic ganglia. The ganglion then transmits sympathetic fibres to the same level via the grey rami communicantes (postganglionic), or may send preganglionic fibres upwards or downwards. Preganglionic fibres may also be sent from the ganglia to a distant collateral ganglion, such as the coeliac plexus or cervical ganglion, or the adrenal medulla. The parasympathetic system is somewhat less well defined and has its outflow from the third, sixth, ninth and tenth cranial nerves as well as S2–4. The ganglia are some distance from the spinal cord and the preganglionic fibres relay close to the end organ. For this reason the postganglionic fibres are necessarily much shorter than in the sympathetic system.

Functionally, the sympathetic nervous system is concerned with the stress reactions of the body ('fight or flight'). The parasympathetic nervous system is concerned with homeostasis and tends to antagonise the sympathetic activity to return the body to its resting state.

## SYMPATHETIC NERVOUS SYSTEM

The sympathetic trunk (ganglionated) extends from the base of skull to the coccyx, in close proximity to the vertebral column. Sympathetic fibres from T1 to L2 synapse in the ganglionic chain at the same level, or ascend or descend to synapse in higher or lower ganglia or plexuses. Somatic sympathetic fibres accompany each spinal nerve (grey rami) to provide sympathetic supply to the skin of the respective dermatome. Visceral fibres supply sympathetic supply to the head, neck and thoracic viscera from specialised ganglia, and the abdominal and pelvic viscera receive fibres from nearby plexuses.

1. Sympathetic ganglia:
   - Cervical ganglia – three:
     - Superior cervical ganglion (C1–4) – sends fibres to the internal and external carotid artery, otic, ciliary and submandibular ganglia, spinal nerve rami and cardiac plexus
     - Middle cervical ganglion (C5 and C6) – sends fibres to the inferior thyroid artery, spinal nerve rami and cardiac plexus

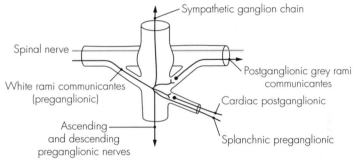

Sympathetic ganglion chain

Spinal nerve

Postganglionic grey rami
communicantes

White rami communicantes
(preganglionic)

Cardiac postganglionic

Ascending
and descending
preganglionic nerves

Splanchnic preganglionic

**Fig 19.1**
Distribution of the (thoracic) sympathetic nerves

- Inferior cervical ganglion (C7 and C8) – sends fibres to the vertebral artery, spinal nerve rami and cardiac plexus. However, in 80% of cases, it is fused with T1 to form the stellate ganglion
- Stellate ganglion – formed from C7 to T1. It has a close anatomical relationship with the lower sympathetic chain. It is positioned anterior and between the transverse process of T7 and the first rib, and lies behind the vertebral artery. Stellate ganglion blockade may be performed with the head in full extension. The transverse process of C7 is usually easily palpated with firm pressure 3 cm above the sternoclavicular joint. The needle is inserted at right angles to the skin, and with the sternomastoid muscle and carotid artery retracted laterally, the transverse process is met ~3 cm from the skin. The local anaesthetic is then injected, after careful aspiration
- Thoracic ganglia – usually 12. They supply fibres to the aorta, spinal nerve rami, three splanchnic nerves (greater, lesser, lowest) and the cardiac, pulmonary and oesophageal plexuses
- Lumbar ganglia – usually four. Branches go to the aortic and hypogastric plexuses, and lumbar spinal nerves
- Sacral ganglia – four. Supply pelvic plexuses and sacral spinal nerves
2. Sympathetic plexuses:
   - Cardiac plexus:
     - Deep cardiac plexus lies in front of the tracheal bifurcation and receives branches from the cervical and upper four thoracic ganglia as well as the vagal branches
     - Superficial cardiac plexus lies anterior to the pulmonary artery and under the aortic arch. It receives the upper right cervical ganglion branches and the left vagus lower cardiac branch
   - Coeliac plexus – largest sympathetic plexus. It is found as a dense network of fibres anterior to the aorta, around the origin of the coeliac artery (at L1). It lies behind the superior border of the pancreas and the stomach. It receives the greater, lesser and lowest splanchnic nerves and the coeliac branch of the right vagus. Some fibres relay directly to the adrenal medulla, and the remainder descend down the aorta to form the aortic plexus. The celiac plexus may be also be blocked, usually with the patient prone. A long spinal needle is inserted ~6 cm from the midline, at the lower costal margin. The needle is angled towards the first lumbar vertebral body and 'slipped off' anteriorly for a short distance. Careful aspiration should precede the injection (the aortic pulsation can frequently be felt)
   - Hypogastric plexus – lies on the sacral promontory between the common iliac arteries. It receives the presacral nerves (from lumbar trunks and aortic plexus) and the sympathetic nerves spread further to the pelvis plexuses

## PARASYMPATHETIC NERVOUS SYSTEM

The parasympathetic nervous system has cranial and sacral components:

1. Cranial – conveyed in cranial nerves III, VII, IX and X. The functions

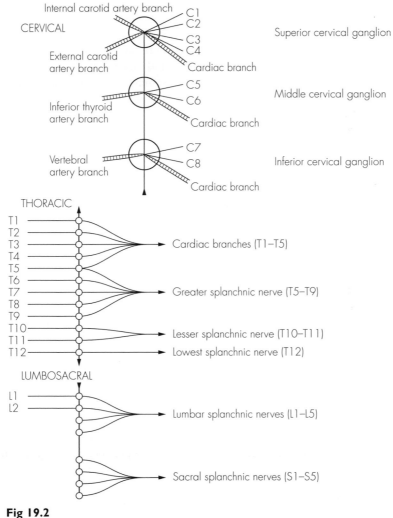

**Fig 19.2**
The sympathetic outflow

are, briefly, pupillary constriction, accommodation, salivary and lacrimal secretomotor, cardiac inhibition, bronchoconstriction and intestinal motor activity:

- III nerve (oculomotor) – relays in the ciliary ganglion
- VI nerve (facial) – relays in the pterygopalatine and submandibular ganglia
- IX nerve (glossopharyngeal) – relays in the otic ganglion
- X nerve (vagus) – most important parasympathetic outflow. The efferent fibres come from the dorsal nucleus of the vagal medullary nucleus and distribute widely to the cardiac, pulmonary and abdominal plexuses

2. Sacral – formed from the ventral primary rami of S2–4 and form the pelvic splanchnic nerves. These join the sympathetic plexuses to then relay in tiny end-organ ganglia. Functionally, the fibres provide rectal and bladder motor function, inhibit sphincteric muscle and cause genital vasodilation

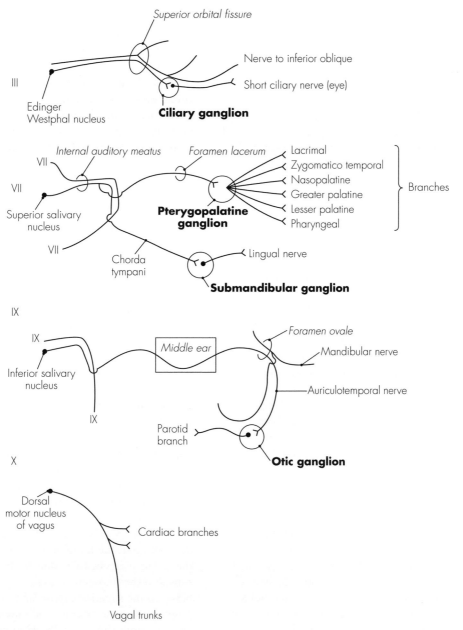

**Fig 19.3**
The parasympathetic outflow

# 20    The cranial nerves

The cranial nerves can be thought of as the peripheral nerves of the brain. These originate from cranial nerve nuclei, which are situated in the pons and medulla (the embryological hindbrain). There are 12 cranial nerves, of which two are somewhat atypical: the olfactory nerve (formed by extended olfactory sensory processes) and optic nerve (a tract drawn out from the brain during development).

1.  Olfactory nerve (I) – consists of an olfactory tract with direct connections to the anterior part of the brain. The cribriform plate allows the olfactory sensory cells to pass through, and these synapse with the olfactory bulb. The bulb leads to the olfactory tract, which runs on the inferior surface of the frontal lobe

2.  Optic nerve (II) – fibres pass from the retina via the optic disc to the optic nerve. This passes through the orbit within the muscle cone, and goes through the optic foramen (in the sphenoid bone), above the ophthalmic artery, into the middle cranial fossa. Here it lies medial to the anterior clinoid process before running laterally and then superior to the sella turcica. The optic chiasma is formed here, with the temporal fields crossing to the opposite side. The nerves continue on each side between the temporal uncus and the cerebral peduncle to reach the lateral geniculate body (in the thalamus). Some fibres also extend to reach the superior colliculus, subserving the ocular and papillary reflexes. The lateral geniculate body then sends fibres via the optic radiation to the occipital cortex

3.  Oculomotor nerve (III) – emerges medial to the cerebral peduncle to reach the middle cranial fossa. It then runs forward, close to the posterior communicating artery, and pierces the dura to enter the cavernous sinus superiorly and laterally. It descends medial to the trochlear nerve and enters the orbit within the tendinous ring and through the superior orbital fissure. It divides into two divisions:
    - Superior – supplying superior rectus and levator palpebrae superioris
    - Inferior – supplying medial rectus, inferior rectus and inferior oblique
    In addition to the above muscular supply, the oculomotor nerve also carries preganglionic fibres (to pupillary sphincter and ciliary muscle) from the Edinger–Westphal parasympathetic nucleus. These relay in the ciliary ganglion situated in the lateral orbit

4.  Trochlear nerve (IV) – emerges (after decussating in the midbrain) lateral to the superior cerebellar peduncle. It runs into the mid-cranial fossa, between the superior cerebellar and posterior cerebral arteries, and enters the cavernous sinus laterally. Here it lies below, and is crossed medially by, the III nerve. It runs through the superior orbital fissure and terminates by supplying the superior oblique muscle

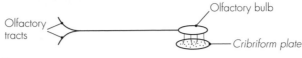

**Olfactory nerve**

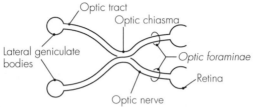

**Optic nerve**

**Fig 20.1**
The olfactory and optic nerves

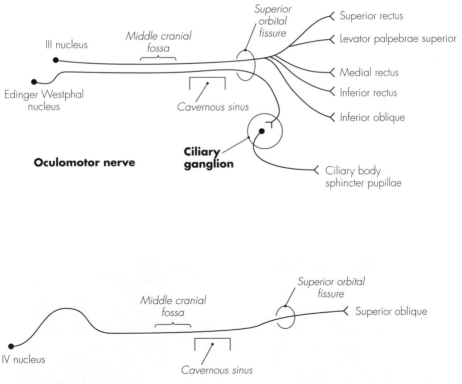

**Oculomotor nerve**

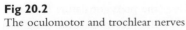

**Trochlear nerve**

**Fig 20.2**
The oculomotor and trochlear nerves

5.  Trigeminal nerve (V) – largest cranial nerve. It has a small motor and a large sensory root and is associated with four autonomic ganglia. It is responsible for the majority of sensory supply to the face, nose, mouth and orbit, and supplies motor fibres to the muscles of mastication, posterior digastric, mylohyoid, tensor palati and tensor tympani. It also communicates with the ciliary, pterygopalatine, submandibular and otic ganglia. The motor nucleus is situated in the upper pons, just below the floor of the fourth ventricle. The sensory nucleus is divided into three parts: mesencephalic (high mid-brain), superior (upper pons) and spinal tract (runs parallel to the pons and medulla nuclei). These nuclei each subserve different sensory inputs. The combined roots of the trigeminal nerve emerge from the ventrolateral aspect of the pons. The larger lateral sensory root develops a swelling after 1 cm – the trigeminal ganglion:

    - Trigeminal ganglion – lies near the apex of the petrous temporal bone (slightly hollowed). The motor root of the trigeminal nerve runs beneath it, above it lies the temporal lobe. Medially lie the posterior cavernous sinus and internal carotid artery. Fibres pass posteriorly below the superior petrosal sinus to reach the pons, and anteriorly the nerve divides into three divisions: ophthalmic, maxillary and mandibular divisions. During local nerve blockade of the ganglion, the needle is introduced below the posterior zygomatic bone and behind the pterygoid plate. The foramen ovale is located radiologically, and the needle advanced through this to a further depth of 1 cm. Dural puncture is possible and careful aspiration is required, prior to injection

The three divisions of the trigeminal nerve are:

- Ophthalmic nerve – smallest of the three divisions. It provides sensation only to the superior face and anterior scalp. Prior to entering the orbit, the ophthalmic nerve divides into three branches – all of which pass through the superior orbital fissure:

    Frontal nerve – divides into the supra-orbital nerve (supplies the upper eyelid and scalp) and supratrochlear nerve (supplies the skin of the forehead)

    Nasociliary nerve – branches are long ciliary nerves (eyeball), ganglionic (ciliary), ethmoidal nerves (ethmoid and nasal cavity) and infratrochlear nerve (lacrimal sac and eyelid)

    Lacrimal nerve – supplies the lacrimal gland and upper eyelid

- Maxillary nerve – also purely sensory, to the mid-facial region. It passes through the foramen rotundum into the pterygopalatine fossa and via the fissure into the infratemporal fossa. It exits through the inferior orbital fossa and continues as the infra-orbital nerve. The maxillary nerve has numerous branches during its course:

    Meningeal branches – within the cranium (dura mater)

    Ganglionic branches – within the pterygopalatine fossa (to the pterygopalatine ganglion)

    Zygomatic nerve – within the pterygopalatine fossa into

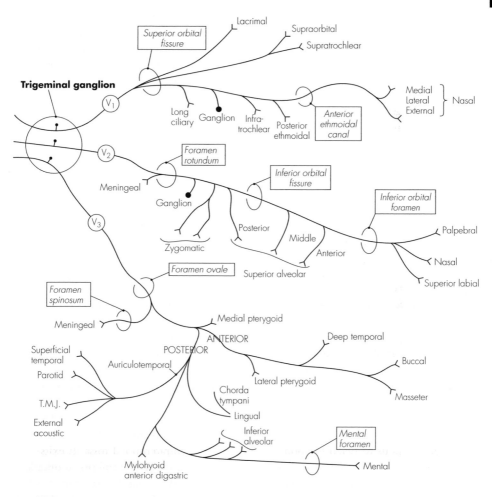

**Fig 20.3**
The trigeminal nerve

two branches (-facial and -temporal – to the cheek and temple)

Posterior superior alveolar nerve – within the pterygopalatine fossa (to the maxillary sinus, maxillary molar, cheek and gums)

Middle superior alveolar nerve – from the infra-orbital nerve (to the maxillary sinus and upper premolar tooth)

Anterior superior alveolar nerve – from the infra-orbital nerve (to the maxillary sinus and canine and incisor teeth)

Infra-orbital nerve (terminal) – divides into the palpebral, nasal and superior labial branches

- Mandibular nerve – sensory and motor. The nerve exits through the foramen ovale and gives off two branches (sensory to the dura mater, motor to the medial pterygoid muscle), before bifurcating into the anterior (small) and posterior (large) trunks:

Anterior trunk – gives off:
  Buccal nerve (sensory to the cheek)
  Masseteric nerve (motor to the masseter)
  Deep temporal nerves (motor to the temporalis)
  Nerve to lateral pterygoid

Posterior trunk – gives off:
  Auriculotemporal nerve (five terminal branches supply the acoustic meatus and ear fibres, temporomandibular joint, temporal skin and parotid parasympathetic)
  Lingual nerve (joined by the chorda tympani (VII), sensory to the mucous membrane of the mouth, tongue and gums)
  Inferior alveolar nerve (lower teeth and gums, then through the mental foramen to supply the lower lip/chin, also gives off the nerve to the mylohyoid)

6. Abducent nerve (VI) – emerges from the lower border of the pons and crosses the pontine basal cistern before piercing the dura inferolateral to the sella turcica. Arching over the petrous temporal bone, it runs on the medial wall of the cavernous sinus and lateral to the internal carotid artery. It enters the orbit through the superior orbital fissure to supply the lateral rectus muscle

7. Facial nerve (VII) – mixed nerve with complex arrangements. It supplies motor fibres to the muscles of expression, carries parasympathetic innervation to the salivary, palatine and lacrimal glands, taste from the anterior two-thirds of the tongue and sensation to the external auditory meatus, tympanic membrane and ear. It emerges from the pontomedullary junction as two roots – a visceral efferent root and a mixed nervus intermedius. It runs (together with the VIIIth nerve) into the internal auditory meatus (in the posterior petrous bone), and runs in the facial canal and then in the lateral middle ear. A sharp bend in the tortuous course of the facial nerve (at the medial wall between the inner and middle ear) marks the site of the geniculate (facial) ganglion. The nerve continues down in the tympanic cavity posteriorly and exits through the stylomastoid foramen. After winding laterally around the styloid process, the facial nerve dives into the posterior part of the parotid

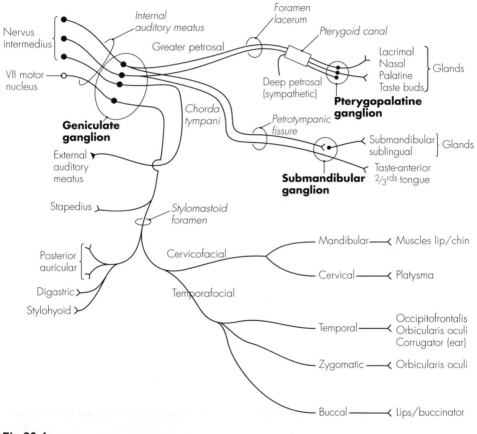

**Fig 20.4**
The facial nerve

gland and divides into two divisions (cervicofacial and temporofacial). The facial nerve has the following branches:

- Greater petrosal nerve – emerges from the geniculate ganglion (and contains the lacrimal secretomotor fibres) to run underneath the trigeminal ganglion, and then forwards to join the pterygopalatine ganglion
- Chorda tympani – branches off prior to the facial nerve leaving the stylomastoid foramen. It runs along the tympanic membrane and exits from the middle ear anteriorly through the petrotympanic fissure. It joins the lingual nerve and conveys secretomotor fibres to the submandibular ganglion and taste from the anterior two-thirds of the tongue
- Muscular fibres – after exiting the stylomastoid foramen, the facial nerve is entirely motor:
  - Posterior auricular – to the extrinsic ear muscles and occipitofrontalis
  - Digastric branch – to the posterior digastric
  - Stylohyoid branch – to the stylohyoid muscle
- Cervicofacial division – has two branches. The mandibular branch supplies the lower lip and chin muscles, the cervical branch supplies platysma
- Temporofacial division – usually has three branches. The temporal branches supply the ear muscle, occipitofrontalis and orbicularis oculi. The zygomatic branches also supply the orbicularis oculi. The buccal branches supply the lips and buccinator

8. Vestibulocochlear nerve (VIII) – also called the auditory nerve. This emerges from the cerebellopontine angle as a single nerve. It enters the internal auditory meatus, where the cochlear part separates and pierces the temporal bone (to supply the cochlear modiolus). The vestibular portion also pierces the temporal bone after dividing into two upper and lower divisions (to supply the semicircular canals, utricle and saccule)

9. Glossopharyngeal nerve (IX) – mixed nerve derived from four cranial nuclei. These are the rostral part of nucleus ambiguous, the inferior salivatory nucleus, the tractus solitarius and the dorsal sensory nucleus. The nerve emerges from the upper medulla as a number of rootlets (four or five). It runs in a groove between the inferior cerebellar peduncle and the olive, and descends to leave the skull through the jugular foramen. It then runs between the internal jugular vein and internal carotid artery before curving anteriorly, and enters the pharynx between the superior and middle constrictors. The supply is:
- Superior and inferior ganglion – within the jugular foramen, serve as relay stations
- Tympanic branch – supplies the tympanic cavity and continues as the lesser petrosal nerve (parasympathetic) to the otic ganglion (parotid secretomotor)
- Carotid nerve – runs down the internal carotid artery and supplies the carotid sinus (pressor) and body (chemo)
- Terminal branches – contribute to the pharyngeal plexus and supply sensation to the tonsils, pharynx, soft palate and posterior one-third of the tongue

10. Vagus nerve (X) – large and widely distributed cranial nerve. It arises

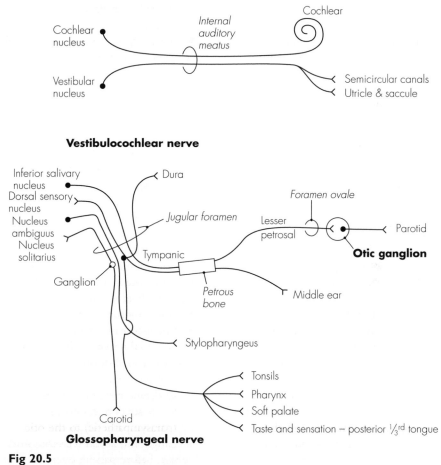

**Vestibulocochlear nerve**

**Glossopharyngeal nerve**

**Fig 20.5**
The vestibulocochlear and glossopharyngeal nerves

from three cranial nuclei: dorsal
nucleus of vagus, nucleus ambiguus
and nucleus of the tractus solitarius. It
emerges from the upper medulla
alongside the glossopharyngeal nerve
as a set of rootlets (nine or ten), and
continues similarly in the
posterolateral groove. The vagus soon
forms a single trunk and exits the
skull through the jugular foramen.
Two small ganglia are present on the
vagus nerve within the jugular
foramen: superior (with cell bodies
from the ear and dura) and inferior
(other afferents). The cranial part of
the accessory nerve fuses with the
vagus just below the jugular foramen.
The distal course of the vagus nerve
differs somewhat on each side. Both
vagi descend within the carotid
sheath and lie in front of the cervical
sympathetic chain. On the right, the
vagus descends in front of the right
subclavian artery and gives off the
right recurrent laryngeal nerve.
Passing behind the right
brachiocephalic vein, it descends into
the thorax against the trachea and
behind the root of the right lung. It
gives branches to the right posterior
pulmonary and oesophageal plexuses,
and enters the abdomen behind the
oesophageal hiatus. It proceeds to
give branches to the upper stomach
before forming the coeliac branch (to
the coeliac plexus). The left vagus
runs down between the left carotid
and left subclavian artery to pass
behind the left brachiocephalic vein.
It crosses over the aortic arch, giving
off the left recurrent nerve, and
descends into the thorax behind the
left lung root. Branches are also given
to the posterior pulmonary and
oesophageal plexuses, but the nerve
now runs anteriorly and close to the

oesophagus through the oesophageal
hiatus. Apart from branches to the
lower stomach and pylorus, a hepatic
branch is also given off. The branches
of the vagus nerve are:
- In jugular foramen – meningeal
  and auricular branches
- In neck – pharyngeal branch,
  superior laryngeal nerve, right
  recurrent laryngeal nerve and
  cardiac branches
- In thorax – cardiac branches, left
  recurrent laryngeal nerve,
  pulmonary, pericardial and
  oesophageal branches
- In abdomen – gastric, hepatic and
  coeliac branches
11. Accessory nerve (XI) – derived from
two roots, a cranial (from nucleus
ambiguus) and a spinal root (from C1
to C5). After emerging as numerous
rootlets behind the olive, the nerve
fuses with the spinal root (having
ascended through foramen magnum)
and exits the skull through the
jugular foramen. The cranial root
joins the vagus, and the spinal root
descends laterally in front of the atlas
to supply motor fibres to the
sternocleidomastoid and trapezius
12. Hypoglossal nerve (XII) – emerges as
a series of small rootlets from the
anterolateral medulla. These fuse
along their course behind the
vertebral artery and into the
hypoglossal canal. It emerges
anteriorly and laterally to the neck
vessels, before passing over the hyoid
greater cornu, and terminates under
the submandibular gland. The
hypoglossal nerve supplies motor
fibres to the intrinsic muscles of the
tongue, hyoglossus, genioglossus and
styloglossus (as well as receiving fibres
from the cervical ventral rami for
distribution to the neck muscles)

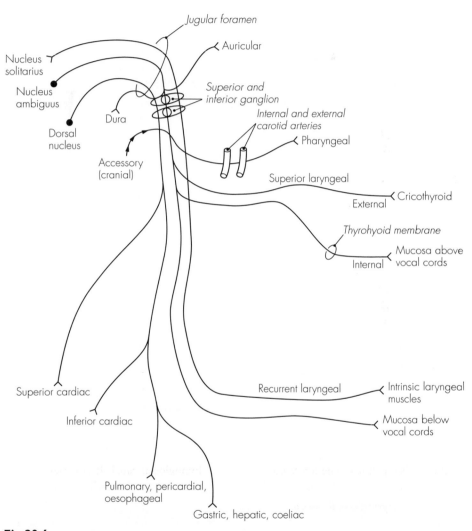

**Fig 20.6**
The vagus nerve

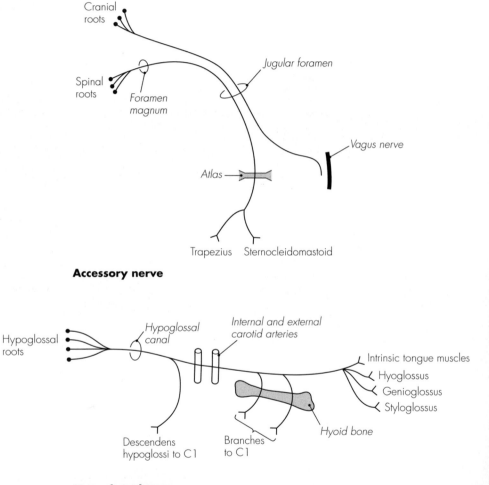

**Accessory nerve**

**Hypoglossal nerve**

**Fig 20.7**
The accessory and hypoglossal nerves

# Appendices

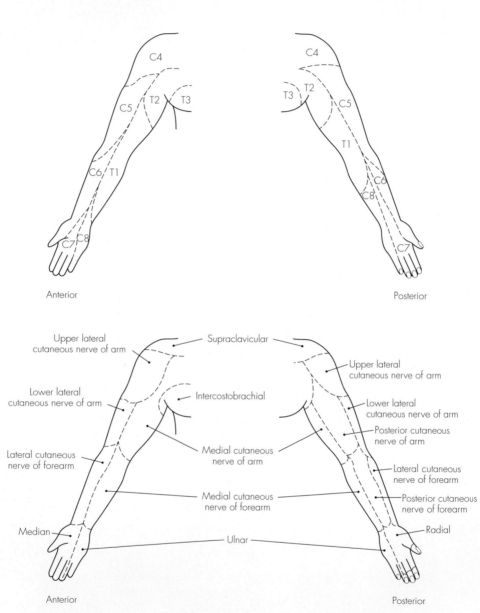

**App I**
Dermatomes and cutaneous nerves of arm

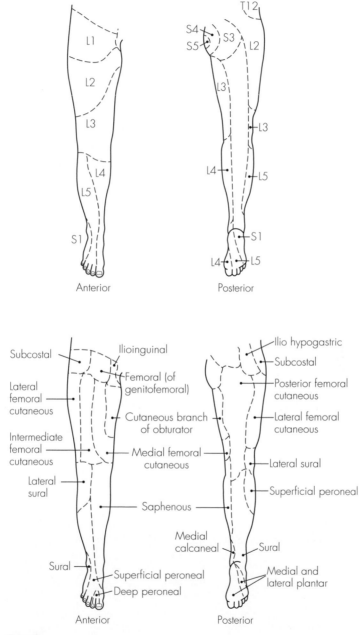

**App 2**
The dermatomes of the leg

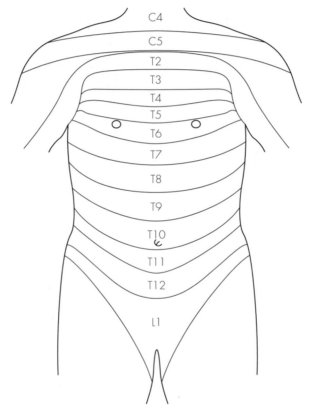

**App 3**
The dermatomes of the trunk

# Sample questions – nervous system

1. Describe, with the aid of a diagram, the blood supply to the brain.
2. Using a simple diagram, detail the path of a typical intercostal nerve from its origin to its terminal branches.
3. What is the nerve supply of the abdominal wall?
4. Draw a cross-sectional labelled diagram of the spinal column to illustrate the relationships of the epidural space.
5. Discuss, in point form, the anatomy of the brachial plexus. Briefly describe one method of performing a brachial plexus nerve block.
6. Describe how you would carry out an axillary brachial plexus nerve block.
7. Draw a labelled diagram of the relations of the stellate ganglion. How is it blocked and what are the possible complications?
8. Describe your technique for a coeliac plexus block with reference to the important anatomical features.
9. How is an ankle block performed? Explain how the sensory innervation of the foot is related to individual nerves.
10. Describe the course of the femoral/sciatic nerve. How do you perform a femoral/sciatic nerve block?
11. Draw a labelled diagram of the anterior aspect of the wrist. How may this knowledge be of use in anaesthetic practice?

# Vertebral Column

# 21   The vertebrae

1. Vertebral column – midline structure extending from the base of the skull above to the pelvis below. It provides protection for the spinal cord and transfers weight through the pelvis, as well as having an extensive area for muscular attachment. It consists of bony vertebrae connected by intervertebral fibrocartilaginous discs
2. Twenty-four true vertebrae – seven cervical, 12 thoracic and five lumbar. There are nine false vertebrae, which consist of the sacrum (five fused vertebrae) and the vestigial coccyx (four fused vertebrae)
3. Vertebral column – also has a number of curved segments. In the adult, there are two areas that are convex anteriorly: cervical and lumbar curvatures. The thoracic and sacral areas show anteriorly concave curvatures

## DESCRIPTION

A typical vertebra has an anterior body and a posterior neural arch. The lumbar bodies are the largest, having to support proportionately more weight. The vertebral bodies are each separated by a tough fibrocartiligenous disc. The neural arch is connected to the vertebral body by two strong pedicles of bone. The pedicles each have articular facets (superior and inferior), which articulate with similar facets of the adjacent vertebra as a synovial joint (facet joint). The neural arch is completed posteriorly by the two bony laminae joining to form a spinous process. A transverse process on each side projects laterally and provides additional surface area for muscular attachment. There are also two costal processes on each vertebral body, which are well developed in the thoracic area. The detailed structure of the individual vertebrae varies considerably:

Cervical vertebrae – the typical cervical vertebra is found from C3 to C6. It has a relatively small and wide body, and has two lateral processes (for the synovial joints of Lushka) on the superior surface of the body. The transverse processes also contain a foramen (transversarium) for the passage of the vertebral artery, venous and sympathetic plexuses. The spinal nerve exits from the vertebral column via a shallow neural groove, between the anterior and posterior tubercle of the transverse processes. The laminae are flat and long, and terminate in bifid spinous processes (often single at C6). The neural canal is roughly triangular in cross-section and widest at C5. The atypical cervical vertebrae are:

- Atlas (C1) – has no true body and essentially consists of a ring of bone. It supports the weight of the skull and articulates with the occipital condyles on its superior articular facets. The inferior facets articulate with the axis below. It also has a rounded facet on the anterior arch for articulation with the odontoid peg of the axis. The skull rocks backward and forward on the atlas

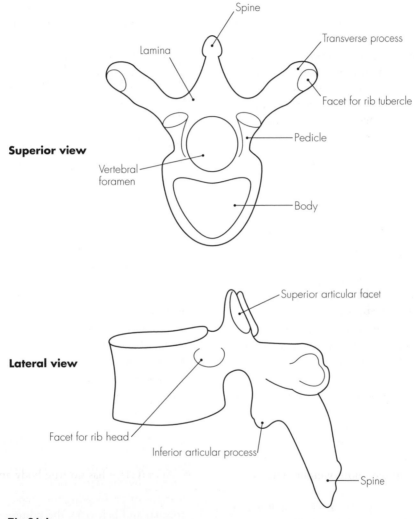

**Superior view**

Spine

Lamina

Transverse process

Facet for rib tubercle

Pedicle

Vertebral
foramen

Body

**Lateral view**

Superior articular facet

Facet for rib head

Inferior articular process

Spine

**Fig 21.1**
A typical vertebra

- Axis (C2) – allows the head to rotate. It is also somewhat ring-like in shape. It has a projection of bone from the body – odontoid peg or dens, which is attached to the occipital bone by apical ligaments. The laminae are particularly strong and the transverse processes short
- Vertebra prominens (C7) – largest cervical vertebra. It has a particularly large spinous process and is transitional between the cervical and thoracic vertebrae. Occasionally, a cervical rib may also be seen, extending from the transverse process

Thoracic vertebrae – have articular facets on the vertebral bodies and transverse processes for articulation with the head and neck of the rib. The vertebral bodies are somewhat heart-shaped and have lateral half-facets (superiorly and inferiorly) for the articulation of the head of the rib. The transverse processes are directed backwards and laterally, and carry facets on the anterior aspect for articulation with the tubercle of the rib. The spinous processes are generally slender, long and are directed caudad. The atypical vertebrae are:

- T1 – similar to C7, with a broader and wider body. The upper costal facet is complete for articulation with the first rib and a transverse process facet placed more anteriorly. An articular shelf is also present, providing additional support to prevent backward displacement of C7 on T1
- T9 and T10 – may only show single costal articular facets
- T11 and T12 – transitional between the thoracic and lumbar vertebrae (being stronger and having smaller transverse processes)

Lumbar vertebrae – largest vertebrae and lack foramina transversaria and costal facets. The bodies are large and kidney-shaped, the pedicles short and strong, and the transverse processes relatively small. The superior and inferior articular facets are vertically orientated. The body of L5 is wedge-shaped – thicker posteriorly than anteriorly.

Sacrum – formed by the fusion of the five sacral vertebrae. It forms the central axis of the pelvic girdle, and articulates above with the fifth lumbar vertebra, on the sides with the innominate bone (at the sacroiliac joints), and below with the coccyx. It is concave anteriorly and roughly wedge-like in shape, and has four pairs of foramina for the exit of the ventral spinal nerves posteriorly.

The sacral canal is within the sacrum, with anterior and posterior margins created by the fused sacral vertebrae. It contains:
- Cauda equina
- Filum terminale
- Meninges (spinal)
- Coccygeal/sacral nerves
- Epidural fat and veins

The lower part of the sacrum shows that the fifth sacral laminae frequently fail to fuse. This is called the sacral hiatus. The hiatus is bounded above by the fused fourth sacral laminae, laterally by the deficient lamina margins of S5 (bearing the sacral cornua) and below by the posterior body of S5.

The hiatus is covered over by the sacrococcygeal ligament, and this provides a convenient entry route into the caudal epidural space. The cornua are identified with a fingertip, and a needle introduced at 45° to the skin. Once the sacral canal is entered, the

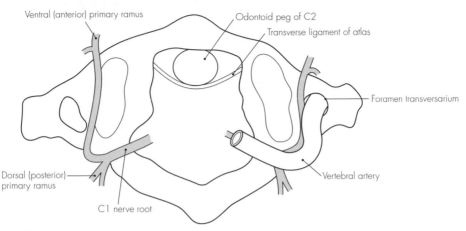

Ventral (anterior) primary ramus

Odontoid peg of C2

Transverse ligament of atlas

Foramen transversarium

Dorsal (posterior) primary ramus

Vertebral artery

C1 nerve root

**Fig 21.2**
The atlas (C1)

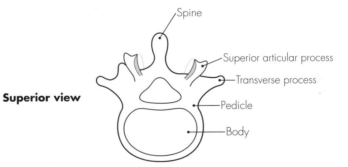

Spine

Superior articular process

Transverse process

Pedicle

Body

**Superior view**

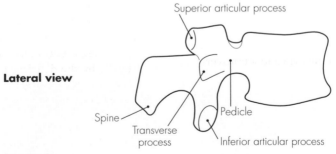

Superior articular process

Spine

Pedicle

Transverse process

Inferior articular process

**Lateral view**

**Fig 21.3**
A lumbar vertebra

needle is advanced a short distance and the solution injected. Care must be taken to avoid entering the subdural space, especially in children where the dural sac may end unusually low.

Coccyx – formed from the fusion of four small and rudimentary coccygeal vertebrae. The surfaces provide attachment for nearby pelvic and gluteal muscles

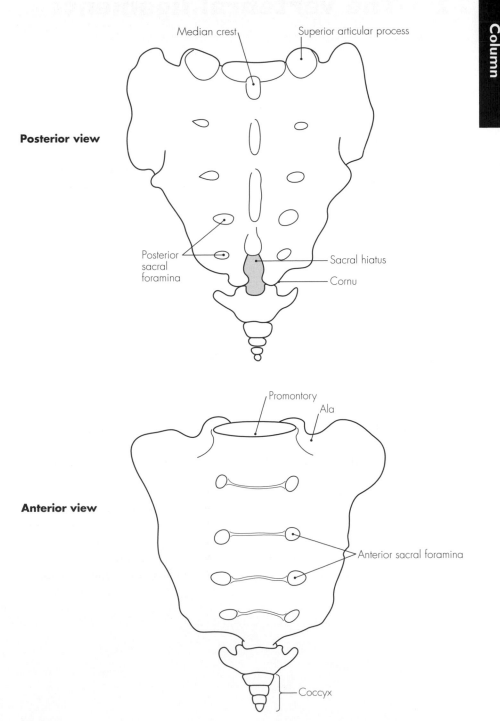

**Posterior view**

Median crest

Superior articular process

Posterior
sacral
foramina

Sacral hiatus

Cornu

**Anterior view**

Promontory

Ala

Anterior sacral foramina

Coccyx

**Fig 21.4**
The sacrum and coccyx

# 22    The vertebral ligaments

## DESCRIPTION

There is a complicated series of ligaments and joints that connect the various components of the vertebral column. These may be summarised as follows:

Intervertebral discs – connect the vertebral bodies and make up 25% of the height of the spinal column. These consist of an outer annulus fibrosus and an inner annulus pulposus. The superior and inferior surfaces of the vertebral bodies are also lined with hyaline cartilage, which allow adhesion to the intervertebral discs

Anterior longitudinal ligament – runs along the anterior surface of the vertebral bodies, from C2 to the sacrum. It adheres to the anterior surface of the vertebral bodies and the discs

Posterior longitudinal ligament – extends along the posterior aspect of the vertebral bodies and discs

Ligamenta flava – series of thick, elastic, vertical fibres that connect adjacent vertebral laminae

Interspinous ligaments – connect the shafts of the spinous processes

Supraspinous ligaments – tough fibrous column that connects the tips of the spinous processes

Ligamentum nuchae – superior extension of the supraspinous ligaments and extends from C7 to the occiput

## POINTS OF INTEREST

- The epidural space may be entered by inserting a needle between the spinal vertebral laminae, either directly in the midline, or via a para-midline approach. The needle will pass thorough the following structures as it advances:
  - Skin
  - Subcutaneous tissue and fat
  - Supraspinous ligaments (tough)
  - Interspinous ligaments (thin)
  - Ligamentum flavum (tough)
  - Epidural space (and contents)

# Sample questions – vertebral column

1. Describe the anatomical structures though which the spinal needle passes during a lumbar puncture.
2. How do you perform a caudal block? Detail the important relations of the caudal canal with the aid of a simple diagram.
3. Draw and label a cross-sectional diagram of the epidural space.

# Areas of Special Interest

# 23    The base of the skull

The skull provides protection to the intracranial contents and the face, and consists of the neurocranium and anterior facial (splanchnocranium) structures. The brain rests on the base of the skull, which itself can be divided into three areas or cranial fossae: posterior, middle and anterior.

1.  Posterior cranial fossa – largest and deepest fossa. The sphenoid, temporal and basi-occipital bones bound it anteriorly, and the occipital bone laterally and posteriorly. Posteriorly, the transverse sinuses create deep grooves, which pass laterally, and the occipital prominence lies centrally. This extends to form the internal occipital crest, which attaches to the falx cerebelli. The posterior fossa houses the medulla, pons and cerebellum below and the occipital lobes above (separated by the horizontal tentorium cerebelli). The following openings transmit various structures:
    *   Internal acoustic meatus – situated in the posterior petrous part of the temporal bone, and transmits the facial and vestibulocochlear nerves and labyrinthine vessels
    *   Jugular foramen – lies just below the internal auditory meatus. It transmits the sigmoid and inferior petrosal sinuses, and the glossopharyngeal, vagus and accessory nerves
    *   Hypoglossal canal – transmits the hypoglossal nerve and meningeal branches of the ascending

pharyngeal artery. It lies just anterior to the foramen magnum
    *   Foramen magnum – largest skull opening and transmits the medulla oblongata and meninges, as well as the vertebral arteries and the spinal accessory nerve

2.  Middle cranial fossa – houses the temporal lobes of the brain. It is bounded by the wings of the sphenoid bone anteriorly, the temporal bone laterally, and the petrous temporal crests posteriorly. The sphenoid body houses the hypophyseal fossa centrally (for the pituitary gland) and has two small posterior clinoid processes for attachment to the tentorium cerebelli. The middle cranial fossa communicates with the orbit through two structures: optic canal and the superior orbital fissure. These and other openings transmit the following structures:
    *   Optic canal – placed anteriorly, this transmits the optic nerve and ophthalmic artery
    *   Superior orbital fissure – transmits all the other structures from the orbit
    *   Ophthalmic nerve
    *   Oculomotor, trochlear and abducens nerves
    *   Ophthalmic veins
    *   Foramen rotundum – lies anteriorly in the greater wing of the sphenoid bone. It transmits the maxillary division of the trigeminal nerve
    *   Foramen ovale – placed just

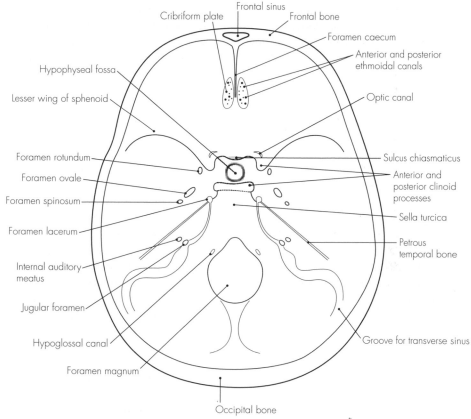

Cribriform plate
Frontal sinus
Frontal bone
Foramen caecum
Anterior and posterior ethmoidal canals
Hypophyseal fossa
Optic canal
Lesser wing of sphenoid
Foramen rotundum
Sulcus chiasmaticus
Foramen ovale
Anterior and posterior clinoid processes
Foramen spinosum
Foramen lacerum
Sella turcica
Petrous temporal bone
Internal auditory meatus
Jugular foramen
Hypoglossal canal
Groove for transverse sinus
Foramen magnum
Occipital bone

**Fig 23.1**
The base of the skull

behind the foramen rotundum and transmits the mandibular division (trigeminal), and the lesser petrosal nerve

- Foramen spinosum – placed further posterolateral to the above, and contains the middle meningeal vessels, and the meningeal branch of the mandibular nerve
- Foramen lacerum – at the junction between the sphenoid and temporal bones posteriorly. It transmits small meningeal branches (of ascending pharyngeal artery) and emissary veins
- Carotid canal – allows the internal carotid artery (and accompanying sympathetic plexus) entrance to the cranium. The artery runs through its large intracranial opening to run anteriorly and medially, lateral to the sphenoid body
- Stylomastoid foramen – has an opening only present on the underside of the skull base. This transmits the facial nerve and branch of the posterior auricular artery and these enter the facial canal

3. Anterior cranial fossa – houses the frontal lobes and is bounded by the frontal bone anteriorly and the lesser wings of sphenoid posteriorly. The floor of the fossa is made of the ethmoid bone centrally and this has a projection – the crista galli – for the attachment to the falx cerebri. The lesser wings of the sphenoid project laterally and terminate medially in the anterior clinoid processes (attach to the tentorium cerebelli). Between the anterior clinoid processes is a slightly indented plateau of bone upon which the optic chiasma lies (sulcus chiasmatus). The following openings are present:

- Foramen caecum – anterior to the crista galli and transmits an emissary vein
- Cribriform plate – transmits the olfactory sensory nerves
- Anterior ethmoidal canal – just lateral to the cribriform plate and for the passage of anterior ethmoidal nerves and vessels
- Posterior ethmoidal canal – for the posterior ethmoidal vessels

# 24    The thoracic inlet

The thoracic inlet is the area where the neck and thorax meet, and is filled with a large number of important structures. It is roughly kidney-shaped and is bounded by the superior manubrium anteriorly, the anterior surface of the first vertebral body posteriorly, and the first ribs and cartilages laterally. The lung apices project above the clavicle for ~3 cm, covered over by the pleura and the suprapleural membrane. The lungs are grooved anteriorly by the subclavian vessels and posteriorly by the stellate ganglion, superior intercostal artery and the first thoracic ventral nerve ramus.

The scalenus muscles and the first rib are useful structures to understand the relationships in this area:

1.  Scalenus muscles – three: scalenus anterior, scalenus medius and scalenus posterior. The scalenus anterior originates from the anterior tubercles of C3–6, and passes down and laterally, to attach to the scalene tubercle of the first rib. It lies behind the sternomastoid muscle. The following structures are related to the scalenus anterior:
    *   Anteriorly:
        *   Phrenic nerve
        *   Thoracic duct (on left)
        *   Carotid sheath – superiorly only; inferiorly only the internal jugular vein is anterior (others medial)
        *   Subclavian vein
    *   Posteriorly:
        *   Subclavian artery (divided into parts)
    *   Brachial plexus roots
    *   Medially:
        *   First part of subclavian artery and branches (vertebral, internal thoracic, thyrocervical, costocervical)
        *   Common carotid artery (inferiorly)
        *   Vagus nerve (inferiorly)
        *   Sympathetic trunk

2.  First rib – shortest, flattest and most curved of the ribs. It has a head, a facet for the body of T1, a neck and a tubercle for the transverse process of T1. There are a number of grooves and tubercles on the superior surface of the first rib and these will be described from posterior to anterior:
    *   Insertion for scalenus medius – on the long neck of the first rib and provides for the attachment of the muscle. Immediately in front of the muscle lie the trunks of the brachial plexus
    *   Groove for subclavian artery – just anterior to the scalenus medius muscle groove. It is grooved for the lower trunk of the brachial plexus (posterior) and the subclavian artery (anterior)
    *   Tubercle for scalenus anterior – on the inner medial curve of the first rib, anterior to the subclavian groove
    *   Groove for subclavian vein – just anterior to the insertion of scalenus anterior. The subclavian vein runs over this groove and behind the clavicle

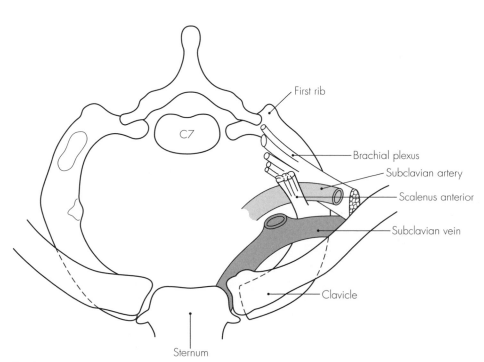

**Fig 24.1**
The thoracic inlet

- Insertion of serratus anterior – on the outer lateral curve of the first rib, opposite the insertion of scalenus anterior

Other structures also attach themselves to the first rib. The suprapleural membrane attaches to the inner margin. The subclavius muscle attaches to the anterior upper extremity. The intercostal muscles attach to the lateral margin.

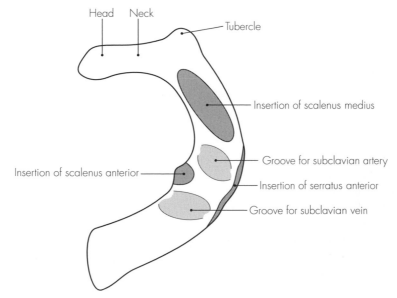

Head    Neck

Tubercle

Insertion of scalenus medius

Groove for subclavian artery

Insertion of scalenus anterior

Insertion of serratus anterior

Groove for subclavian vein

**Fig 24.2**
The first rib

# 25   The intercostal space

The spaces between the ribs are filled by layers of muscle and fibrous tissue, between which are the vessels, nerves and lymphatics.

1. Muscles:
   - External intercostals (11 pairs) – these outermost muscles pass from the lower border of the upper rib to the upper border of the lower rib. They extend anteriorly towards the costochondral junction becoming gradually more fibrous, and merge into the external (anterior) intercostal membrane
   - Internal intercostals (11 pairs) – run deep, and with the fibres running at right angles, to the external intercostals. They extend from the sternum, laterally around to the angle of the rib, where they become fibrous and merge to form the internal (posterior) intercostal membrane
   - Innermost intercostal – largely incomplete and consist of numerous slips of muscle tissue. They are individually named as the transversus thoracis (anteriorly), intracostal (laterally) and subcostalis (posteriorly) muscles. These are bound together by a continuous sheet of fascia. The innermost muscles are also separated from the parietal pleura by a further layer of fascia, the endothoracic fascia
2. Neurovascular bundles – each consist of (from above down) a vein, an artery and a nerve. They lie between the innermost and internal intercostal muscle layers for almost their entire course:
   - Veins – have complex terminations and consist of the posterior and anterior intercostal veins. The posterior veins eventually drain into the superior vena cava via the azygos and hemi-azygos systems, and the anterior veins drain into the musculophrenic vein (lower spaces), or the internal thoracic vein (upper spaces)
   - Arteries – the posterior and anterior intercostal arteries. The posterior intercostal arteries arise directly from the thoracic aorta from T3 to T11, and from the superior intercostal artery (T1 and T2). The anterior intercostal arteries (T1–9) are derived from the two internal thoracic arteries, which themselves are branches of the subclavian artery, and run behind and just lateral to the sternal edge. The last two intercostal spaces are supplied by the posterior intercostal arteries only. The anterior intercostals eventually anastomose with the posterior intercostal arteries
   - Nerves – ventral (anterior) rami of the thoracic nerves from T1 to T11. The lower five nerves from T7 to T11 continue to supply the abdominal wall and maintain their position between the innermost and internal muscle layers (the internal oblique and transversus

abdominus respectively). The typical intercostal nerve has the following branches:

- Rami communicantes – to/from the sympathetic trunk
- Collateral – to the intercostal muscles and pleura
- Lateral cutaneous – to the lateral wall skin and muscles
- Anterior cutaneous – to the anterior wall skin and muscles

Atypically, the first intercostal nerve forms the lower trunk of the brachial plexus, and the second intercostal nerve forms the intercostobrachial nerve (supplies axilla)

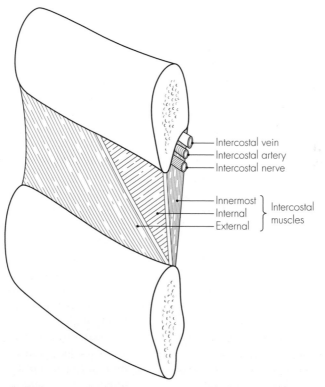

**Fig 25.1**
The intercostal space

# 26    The abdominal wall

This extends from the xiphoid process (at thoracic level T9) and subcostal margin superiorly to the iliac crest, inguinal ligament and pubic symphysis inferiorly. The umbilicus is a convenient central point to divide the abdomen into upper and lower, and right and left, quarters. It is positioned opposite the third lumbar vertebra (and has dermatomal nerve supply from T10). A line joining the iliac crests passes through the body of the fourth lumbar vertebra, and this is also a useful point of reference when performing an epidural or spinal procedure.

The anterior abdominal wall is essentially a layered fibromuscular sheet and has its own blood and nerve supply. Inferiorly, the inguinal region contains numerous structures of importance.

1.  Muscles
    * Rectus abdominus – band-like central pair of muscles arising from the pubic crest and inserting into the fifth, sixth, and seventh costal cartilages. The muscle has at least three horizontal fibrous bands on the anterior surface (preventing easy spread of local anaesthetic solution anteriorly). Each muscle is enclosed by the rectus sheath, which is formed by the splitting of the inferior oblique aponeurosis. This is further reinforced behind by the transversus abdominus aponeurosis and in front by the external oblique aponeurosis. The posterior part of the rectus sheath is deficient superiorly at the costal margin (muscular insertions), and inferiorly below the arcuate line (where the aponeuroses all pass anteriorly to the rectus muscle). In the central region the rectus sheath lies directly on extraperitoneal fat and peritoneum. The rectus sheath contains the rectus abdominus, the superior and inferior epigastric vessels, the terminal branches of the intercostal nerves T7–11, and the subcostal vessels and nerves
    * External oblique – outermost abdominal wall muscle and extends from the lateral edge of the rectus abdominus (linea alba), pubis and anterior iliac crest to the rib insertions. The fibres run downward and medially
    * Internal oblique – lies deep to the external oblique and is continuous with the internal intercostal muscles above. The fibres pass upwards and laterally
    * Transversus abdominus – innermost muscle and its fibres pass horizontally
2.  Blood supply – extensive, and the main supply comes from the inferior epigastric (from the external iliac artery) and superior epigastric (terminal branch of the internal thoracic artery) arteries. The corresponding veins carry the blood away and also lie within the rectus sheath
3.  Nerve supply – from the ventral (anterior) primary rami of T7 to L1. The details of supply have been described earlier.

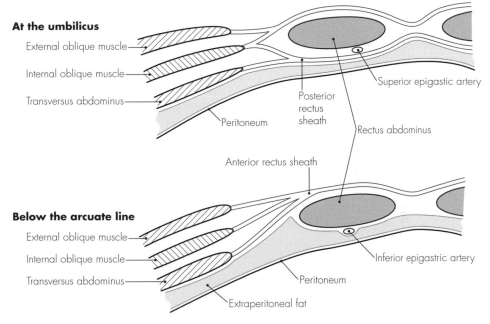

**At the umbilicus**

External oblique muscle

Internal oblique muscle

Transversus abdominus

Peritoneum

Posterior rectus sheath

Superior epigastic artery

Rectus abdominus

Anterior rectus sheath

**Below the arcuate line**

External oblique muscle

Internal oblique muscle

Transversus abdominus

Peritoneum

Inferior epigastric artery

Extraperitoneal fat

**Fig 26.1**
The abdominal wall (cross-section)

# 27 The inguinal region

The inguinal canal is obliquely placed, passing through the lower part of the anterior abdominal wall. It extends from the deep inguinal ring (transversalis fascia opening), down and medially to the superficial ring (external oblique aponeurosis opening). It lies above and follows the inguinal ligament. The inguinal ligament is the rolled-up edge of the external oblique, which runs from the pubic tubercle to the anterior superior iliac spine. The boundaries of the inguinal canal are:

- Anterior – aponeurosis of the external oblique
- Posterior – fascia transversalis, and conjoint tendon in the medial third (common tendon of internal oblique and transversus muscles)
- Floor – inguinal ligament, and lacunar ligament medially
- Roof – arching fibres of the transversus abdominus and internal oblique

The inguinal canal has the following contents:

- Male – ilioinguinal nerve and spermatic cord (containing the vas deferens, testicular, deferens and cremasteric arteries, pampiniform plexus, sympathetic plexus and genital branch of genitofemoral nerve)
- Female – ilioinguinal nerve and round ligament

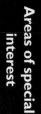

**Superficial**

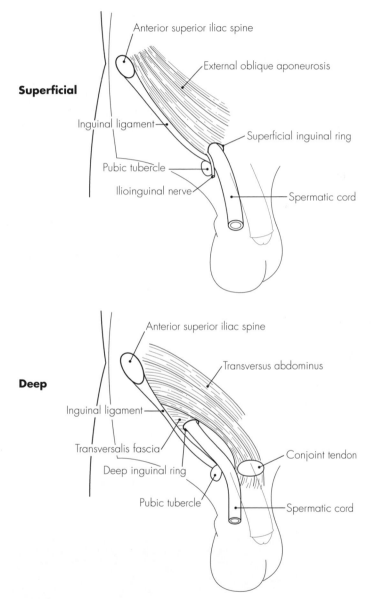

Anterior superior iliac spine

External oblique aponeurosis

Inguinal ligament

Superficial inguinal ring

Pubic tubercle

Ilioinguinal nerve

Spermatic cord

**Deep**

Anterior superior iliac spine

Transversus abdominus

Inguinal ligament

Transversalis fascia

Conjoint tendon

Deep inguinal ring

Pubic tubercle

Spermatic cord

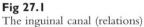

**Fig 27.1**
The inguinal canal (relations)

# 28    The antecubital fossa

## DESCRIPTION

This is the triangular hollowed area on the anterior aspect of the elbow. It contains a number of vessels and nerves that enter and exit the forearm, and which can easily be damaged.

## RELATIONS

Inferomedial – pronator teres
Inferolateral – brachioradialis
Superior – a line joining the two epicondyles of the humerus (medial and lateral)
Roof – deep fascia (reinforced by bicipital aponeurosis). Lying superficial to the fascia are the median cubital vein and the medial cutaneous nerve of the forearm, and the basilic vein (medial) and cephalic vein (lateral)
Floor – supinator (laterally) and brachialis (medially)

## CONTENTS

From medial to lateral:

- Median nerve
- Brachial artery – considerable variations may occur. The artery may bifurcate high in the upper arm, and superficial radial and ulnar branches may also be found. The superficial ulnar artery variation (found in 2%) is at particular risk during antecubital venepuncture attempts
- Biceps tendon
- Radial nerve (with posterior interosseous branch)

## SUPERFICIAL VEINS

These also show considerable variation:

1. Cephalic vein – drains the radial forearm
2. Basilic vein – drains the ulnar forearm
3. Medial cubital vein – joins the basilic and cephalic vein to form an 'H' arrangement. It frequently receives the median vein of the forearm, and may bifurcate to form an 'M' arrangement

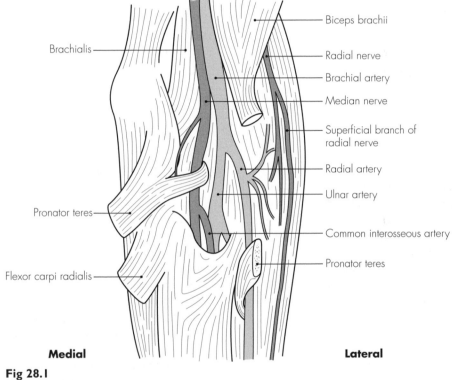

Brachialis

Pronator teres

Flexor carpi radialis

Biceps brachii

Radial nerve

Brachial artery

Median nerve

Superficial branch of radial nerve

Radial artery

Ulnar artery

Common interosseous artery

Pronator teres

**Medial**

**Lateral**

**Fig 28.1**
The antecubital fossa

# 29 The large veins of the neck

These have been briefly discussed earlier, and a more detailed description follows.

1. Internal jugular vein – runs downwards from the jugular foramen (draining the sigmoid sinus) and joins the subclavian vein behind the sternal clavicle to form the brachiocephalic vein. It lies lateral to the internal carotid artery, and lower down, the common carotid artery, within the carotid sheath. The vagus nerve lies just behind and between the two major vessels, within the sheath. The sympathetic chain runs immediately posterior to the carotid sheath and the relations of these two nerves and two vessels are thus similar. The internal jugular vein receives the following tributaries:
   - Pharyngeal veins
   - Common facial vein
   - Thyroid veins (superior and middle)
   - Lingual vein
2. External jugular vein – receives the posterior division of the retromandibular vein (the anterior division joins the facial vein) and crosses anterior to the sternomastoid in the neck. It passes deep to the neck fascia above the clavicle and enters the subclavian vein (not the internal jugular vein)

3. Anterior jugular vein – drains the anterior neck and passes over the thyroid isthmus, diving deep to the sternomastoid, to enter the external jugular vein
4. Subclavian vein – continuation of the axillary vein, and extends from the first rib outer border to the scalenus anterior medial border. It joins the internal jugular vein to form the brachiocephalic vein behind the sternoclavicular joint. It runs over and grooves the first rib in its arch-like course. It also receives the thoracic duct on the left
5. Brachiocephalic vein – formed by the internal jugular and subclavian veins. It receives inferior thyroid, internal thoracic and vertebral veins. The left brachiocephalic vein is 6 cm long and runs behind the manubrium sterni to terminate in forming the superior vena cava (with the right brachiocephalic vein), behind the first costal cartilage. It runs in front of the brachiocephalic artery, trachea and left common carotid artery, and superior to the aortic arch. The right brachiocephalic vein is 3 cm long and runs vertically down behind the right border of the manubrium sterni to form the superior vena cava (as above)

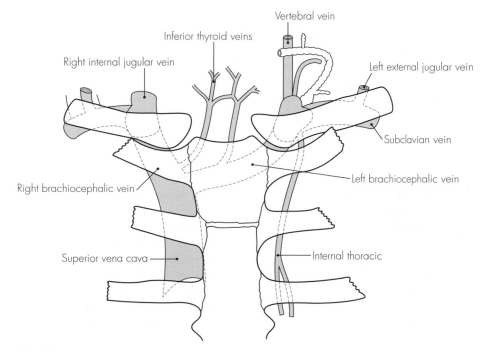

**Fig 29.1**
The large veins of the neck

# 30    The axilla

## DESCRIPTION

This is roughly pyramidal in shape and allows major structures to pass from the neck to the upper limb. The roof extends into the neck and is bounded by the clavicle in front and the scapula behind. The base is bounded by the anterior pectoralis major, the posterior teres major and medially by the chest wall (and serratus anterior muscle), and is covered over by a layer of skin.

## RELATIONS

Anterior wall – pectoralis major and
   minor muscles, and clavipectoral
   fascia
Posterior wall – subscapularis, latissimus
   dorsi and teres major muscles
Medial wall – serratus anterior muscle,
   and upper five ribs and spaces
Lateral wall – coracobrachialis and biceps
   brachii muscles

## CONTENTS

- Axillary artery – continuation of the subclavian artery and becomes the brachial artery at the lower border of teres major. It is invested in a connective tissue sheath – axillary sheath. The pectoralis minor divides the axillary artery into three parts
- Axillary vein – receives the upper limb venous drainage and becomes the subclavian vein. It lies medially along the axillary artery
- Brachial plexus – cords of the brachial plexus surround the axillary artery within the axillary sheath. Initially all cords lie above the axillary artery (in its first part), but take their respective positions (medial, lateral and posterior) in relation to the more distal second part of the artery
- Axillary lymph nodes – these drain the lateral breast and chest wall, and the upper limb. There are six groups that drain into the thoracic duct on the left and the right lymphatic truck on the right

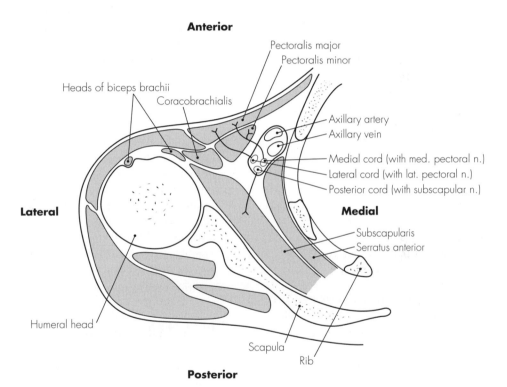

**Anterior**

Pectoralis major
Pectoralis minor

Heads of biceps brachii
Coracobrachialis

Axillary artery
Axillary vein

Medial cord (with med. pectoral n.)
Lateral cord (with lat. pectoral n.)
Posterior cord (with subscapular n.)

**Lateral**

**Medial**

Subscapularis
Serratus anterior

Humeral head

Scapula
Rib

**Posterior**

**Fig 30.1**
The axilla

# 31    The eye and orbit

## DESCRIPTION

The orbit is roughly conical in shape, with the apex directed posteriorly and slightly medially towards the middle cranial fossa. The base is directed towards the face and has strong bony margins to protect the orbital contents. The margins are formed as follows:

Superior – frontal bone (with supra-orbital notch)
Lateral – frontal process of the zygomatic bone
Inferior – frontal process of the zygomatic bone (laterally) and anterior lacrimal crest of the maxilla (medially)
Medial – frontal bone (superiorly), posterior lacrimal crest of the lacrimal bone (inferiorly)

The lacrimal apparatus is contained within a fossa on the medial wall of the orbit, and between the anterior and posterior lacrimal crests.

## RELATIONS

Each orbit has the following boundaries:

Roof – formed from the orbital plate of the frontal bone (anteriorly) and lesser wing of the sphenoid bone (posteriorly). The optic canal is in the posterior roof and transmits the optic nerves, meninges and ophthalmic artery
Medial wall – formed from the orbital lamina of the ethmoid bone, frontal process of the maxilla, lacrimal bone and body of the sphenoid. The lacrimal fossa is formed between the two lacrimal crests on the medial wall. Anterior and posterior ethmoidal foramina on the medial wall transmit ethmoidal nerves and vessels
Floor – formed from the orbital surface of the maxilla and orbital process of the palatine bone. The inferior orbital fissure transmits the infra-orbital artery and nerve
Lateral wall – formed from the frontal process of the zygomatic bone in front and the greater wing of the sphenoid behind. The superior orbital fissure lies between the roof and lateral wall, and transmits the cranial nerves III, IV and VI, the ophthalmic divisions of the trigeminal nerve (V), and the superior ophthalmic vein.

## CONTENTS

- Fat
- Lacrimal apparatus
- Optic nerve
- Orbital vessels
- Eyeball – spherical structure occupying the anterior half of the orbit. It has three coats: an exterior fibrous coat (opaque sclera and transparent cornea), a middle vascular, pigmented coat (choroid, ciliary body and iris), and an inner, delicate, retinal coat. Within the eyeball are the refractive structures: lens, aqueous humour and vitreous body. A thin fascial sheath surrounds the eyeball, except the cornea. This bulbar sheath

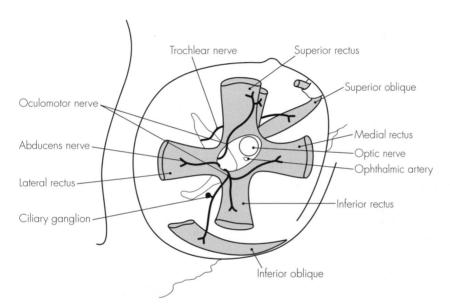

**Fig 31.1**
The eye and orbit

(or Tenon's capsule) separates the eyeball from the surrounding fat and orbital structures. The extra-ocular muscles attach to the corneoscleral junction, and six muscles are responsible for the movement of the eyeball. There are four rectus muscles (medial, lateral, superior, inferior) that arise from a tendinous ring encircling the optic canal and nerve. The two remaining oblique muscles, superior and inferior, arise from the sphenoid bone and orbital surface of the maxilla. Levator palpebrae superioris also arises from the tendinous ring and inserts into and elevates the upper eyelid.

## VASCULAR SUPPLY

1. Arterial:
   - Ophthalmic artery – provides the major blood supply to the orbit and eye. It arises from the internal carotid artery (near the cavernous sinus) and enters the orbit through the optic canal. It gives off a number of branches:
   - Lacrimal artery
   - Posterior ciliary arteries
   - Muscular arteries and anterior ciliary branches
   - Supra-orbital, supratrochlear, nasal and posterior ethmoidal branches
   - Central artery of the retina
2. Venous:
   - Superior ophthalmic vein – passes over the optic nerve and through the superior orbital fissure to terminate in the cavernous sinus. It also anastomoses with the facial vein
   - Inferior ophthalmic vein – passes under the optic nerve and through the inferior orbital fissure to terminate in the superior ophthalmic vein or the cavernous sinus
   - Central vein of the retina – usually passes directly to the cavernous sinus (occasionally joining the superior ophthalmic vein)

## NERVE SUPPLY

May be divided into three groups:
- Motor nerves:
  - Abducens – within the tendinous ring to supply the lateral rectus
  - Trochlear – outside the tendinous ring to supply the superior oblique
  - Oculomotor – inside the tendinous ring to supply other intra-ocular muscles
- Sensory nerves:
  - Optic nerve (as discussed above)
  - Frontal nerve – from the ophthalmic division of the trigeminal nerve to supply the skin of the upper eyelid, forehead and scalp
  - Lacrimal nerve – sensory only to the gland
  - Nasociliary nerve – sensory to the eyeball via numerous branches, including the long and short (also autonomic) ciliary nerves
- Autonomic fibres:
  - Maxillary fibres from the pterygopalatine ganglion – secretomotor to the lacrimal gland
  - Oculomotor nerve – posterior division carries preganglionic parasympathetic fibres to the ciliary ganglion
  - Short ciliary nerves – carry postganglionic fibres from the ciliary ganglion to the sphincter pupillae and ciliary muscles

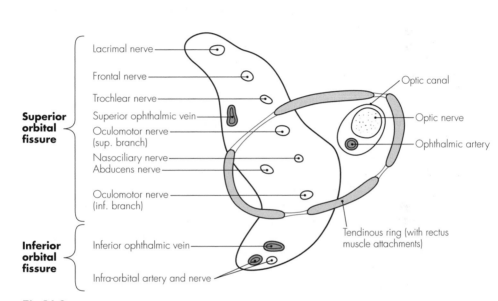

**Superior orbital fissure**
- Lacrimal nerve
- Frontal nerve
- Trochlear nerve
- Superior ophthalmic vein
- Oculomotor nerve (sup. branch)
- Nasociliary nerve
- Abducens nerve
- Oculomotor nerve (inf. branch)

- Optic canal
- Optic nerve
- Ophthalmic artery
- Tendinous ring (with rectus muscle attachments)

**Inferior orbital fissure**
- Inferior ophthalmic vein
- Infra-orbital artery and nerve

**Fig 31.2**
The orbital cone structures

# Sample questions – areas of special interest

1. Using the skull/diagram provided, describe the foraminae marked and list the structures that pass through them.
2. Describe the anatomy of the first rib.
3. What are the important relations and boundaries of the antecubital fossa? What structures may be damaged during attempts at venepuncture in this area?
4. Make a simple diagram, labelled to show the anatomical structures associated with the right jugular vein. List the complications of cannulation of this vessel, mentioning how each may be avoided.
5. Describe the anatomy of the inguinal canal. How may nerve blockade be used to allow surgery under local anaesthesia?
6. What are the bony components of the orbit? Which structures may be damaged during peribulbar and retrobulbar nerve blockade for eye surgery?

# Notes

# Notes

# Notes

# Notes

# Notes

# Notes

# Index

# Index

Note: *a.* = artery/ies; *l.* = ligament/s; *m.* = muscle/s; *n.* = nerve/s; *v.* = vein/s